'You must read Christine Bryden's book if you have any connection with dementia (and even if you do not, because at some point you will). Christine speaks to us elegantly and forcefully from that other "country" of dementia as one of its leading ambassadors. She humanizes this condition, and takes you along on her journey through this territory. No one can truly say that they "understand" dementia until finishing this stirring and totally candid volume. Do so – today.'

– Cameron J. Camp, PhD, Director of Research, Center
for Applied Research in Dementia, Ohio, USA

'Dementia is not a concept, an idea or a diagnostic category. It is a meaningful human experience that occurs within the lives of people who have hopes, dreams and expectations that are not bound by the limitations of failing neurology. In this book, Christine Bryden offers some deep insights into why we need to re-think dementia. Drawing on her own powerful narrative, she offers a way of re-narrating dementia which takes seriously the neurological, but refuses to be defined or reduced to it. As one reflects on the narratives and reflections presented within this book one is inevitably transformed, both in terms of one's thinking about dementia, but more profoundly in terms of realising the breadth and depth of what it actually means to be a human being and to live humanly in all circumstances.'

– Professor John Swinton, Chair in Divinity and Religious Studies, University
of Aberdeen, and author of Dementia: Living in the Memories of God

'*Nothing about us, without us!* demonstrates powerfully that persons with dementia remain persons in the most fundamentally important ways. Christine Bryden, living with dementia for two decades, expertly teaches what helps and what hinders people diagnosed and communicates beautifully why the Golden Rule should be applied regardless of one's medical condition. The book will educate people with dementia, care partners, lay people, and professionals.'

– Steven R. Sabat, PhD, Professor of Psychology, Georgetown
University, author of The Experience of Alzheimer's Disease and
co-editor of Dementia: Mind, Meaning, and the Person

'Christine Bryden speaks and writes with the conviction gained through her experiences of living with and challenging this disease over two decades, since diagnosis. Issues of stigma, care, hope and ways of living effectively with dementia are just some of the important topics she addresses. This collection of talks with slides will form a valuable resource for many: for people who have dementia, for their families, for care providers, and certainly for the wider community.'

– Elizabeth MacKinlay, Centre for Ageing and Pastoral Studies, St Mark's National Theological Centre, School of Theology, Charles Sturt University, Australia

'Dementia is the public health issue of the 21st century. It is the second leading cause of death in Australia, and, in a few short years, will be the leading cause of death of women. *Nothing about us, without us!* questions our automatic responses to dementia, providing a much-needed voice offering inspiration to those who feel "the curse of the pointing-bone of diagnosis". Through personal experience, Christine Bryden identifies misconceptions and prejudices in the way we view and treat people with dementia. People facing a future with dementia will find in this book, an intelligent, positive and authentic voice.'

– James Vickers, Professor of Pathology, University of Tasmania and Chair of the Scientific Panel of the Alzheimer's Australia Dementia Research Foundation

'Christine Bryden, a person of great strength, a survivor with an indestructible spirit, a person living with dementia, invites us to "aspire to a new paradigm of dementia survival with dignity". The book is a chronicle of her life as an advocate who fights each day to retain her dignity and that of all people living with dementia. It is a testament of her consuming passion, to never let go, search for what remains and use it to the maximum. A compelling book for those who seek to better understand what it is like to walk in the shoes of a person with dementia.'

– Frank J. Schaper, Former CEO of Alzheimer's Australia WA Ltd, Alzheimer's Disease International Ambassador and Visiting Fellow of Queensland University of Technology

'Christine Bryden chronicles her two-decade journey living with a diagnosis of dementia, exploding myths and stereotypes along the way. Even in the face of cognitive struggles, Christine embodies personal growth, sharing her insights about the lived experience of dementia. Her inspirational journey of advocacy has evolved to co-founding an international movement on behalf of people who share the diagnosis, and more recently taking on traditional models of care and the need for inclusive communities. I can't wait for the next 20 years!'

– *G. Allen Power, MD, author of* Dementia Beyond Drugs *and* Dementia Beyond Disease

'Christine's journey as a dementia advocate is truly remarkable. This collection of talks and presentations demonstrates the incredible progress that has been made as a result of her determination to make the world a more inclusive place for people living with dementia. I thank Christine for telling her story to the world, and share her hope that this book will help make this dream a reality.'

– *Marc Wortmann, Executive Director, Alzheimer's Disease International*

'Christine Bryden is an inspirational teacher. In this book she takes us through lessons that are deeply honest and simply put, coming from her lived experience and her breath-taking emotional intelligence. This should be compulsory reading for all professionals, people living with dementia and families affected by dementia. There is no us and them. There is only us.'

– *Professor Dawn Brooker, Director of the Association for Dementia Studies, University of Worcester, UK and author of* Person-Centred Dementia Care

NOTHING ABOUT US, WITHOUT US!

by the same author

Dancing with Dementia
My Story of Living Positively with Dementia
Christine Bryden
ISBN 978 1 84310 332 5
eISBN 978 1 84642 095 5

Who will I be when I die?
Christine Bryden
ISBN 978 1 84905 312 9
eISBN 978 0 85700 645 5

of related interest

How We Think About Dementia
Personhood, Rights, Ethics, the Arts and What They Mean for Care
Julian C. Hughes
ISBN 978 1 84905 477 5
eISBN 978 0 85700 855 8

Dementia – Support for Family and Friends
Dave Pulsford and Rachel Thompson
ISBN 978 1 84905 243 6
eISBN 978 0 85700 504 5

Hearing the Person with Dementia
Person-Centred Approaches to Communication for Families and Caregivers
Bernie McCarthy
ISBN 978 1 84905 186 6
eISBN 978 0 85700 499 4

NOTHING ABOUT US, WITHOUT US!

20 years of dementia advocacy

CHRISTINE BRYDEN

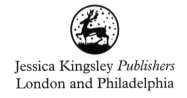

Jessica Kingsley *Publishers*
London and Philadelphia

First published in 2016
by Jessica Kingsley Publishers
73 Collier Street
London N1 9BE, UK
and
400 Market Street, Suite 400
Philadelphia, PA 19106, USA

www.jkp.com

Library of Congress Cataloging in Publication Data
Bryden, Christine, 1949-
Nothing about us, without us! : 20 years of dementia advocacy / Christine Bryden.
pages cm
ISBN 978-1-84905-671-7 (alk. paper)
1. Dementia--Patients--Care. 2. Patient advocacy. I. Title.
RC521.B79 2016
362.1968'3--dc23
2015010226

British Library Cataloguing in Publication Data
A CIP catalogue record for this book is available from the British Library

ISBN 978 1 84905 671 7
eISBN 978 1 78450 176 1

Printed and bound in Great Britain

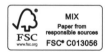

CONTENTS

INTRODUCTION

This book has its genesis in 1995, when I was diagnosed with dementia at the age of only 46. As a recently divorced mother of three girls aged nine, 13 and 19, this was of course a huge shock. Dementia in itself was awful to face, as I had been told I would decline, be in a care home within five years and dead perhaps three years later. However, I also felt isolated by the stigma and fear of society. There was the general perception that dementia was a normal part of ageing, and something either to joke about or to fear: Old Timer's Disease, losing my marbles or the Long Goodbye.

Friends and family seemed to think dementia was simply a bit of memory loss, not a terminal illness that would affect far more than simply my memory, but also finding my way, losing vocabulary and becoming confused. Despite the gloomy future that I faced, and the horror and trauma that I was experiencing, I found that there was no support for people with dementia, only their carers, as we were assumed to lack insight and to be 'mindless empty shells'.

It was these attitudes that made me indignant, outraged, and drove me to become an advocate. I wanted to change these attitudes and to speak out for all those who did not, or could not, speak out on their own behalf. I was featured a few times in the media, and wrote my first book, *Who will I be when I die?*[1] I had 'come out' with my dementia, facing inevitable shame and embarrassment. I found that no one else wanted to admit to having dementia, because everyone treats you differently, tiptoeing around you as if you have become invisible or deaf.

In the same year that this first book was published, I met Paul. We were married in 1999, and he was by my side as I continued my advocacy. I wrote about our love story and these efforts in my second book, *Dancing with Dementia*.[2] With Paul's help, I could face my biggest challenge, which was to persuade the Alzheimer's movement that people with dementia could speak out and be included in these groups that were supposed to be lobbying on our behalf. Only carers were included and listened to at that time. There was a classic Catch 22: we were assumed to be unable to speak if we had dementia, but if we could speak, we did not have dementia. In the face of these prevailing attitudes, I plucked up courage to speak

---

1   Christine Bryden (2012) *Who will I be when I die?* London: Jessica Kingsley Publishers (first published 1998).
2   Christine Bryden (2005) *Dancing with Dementia: My Story of Living Positively with Dementia*. London: Jessica Kingsley Publishers.

at the final session of the Australia Alzheimer's Association Conference in Perth in September 1999, giving an 'inside perspective'.

'Above all,' I said, 'we are individual human beings. We may have a disease. You can't see the damage, but don't assume too much. Take us at face value, as a person first and foremost, not a disease. Then help us to keep on achieving to our full potential.'

The next year, I was delighted to receive an email from Professor Morris Friedell in the US, who had been recently diagnosed with Alzheimer's disease. Morris and I gave a talk, 'Pointing the bone', to the Alzheimer's Australia National Conference, which is included in this book. It made a huge impact and began my collaborative advocacy. By that stage, together with a group of other people with dementia, I had become a founding member of the Dementia Advocacy and Support Network International (DASNI) in 2001. Together we would lobby the global Alzheimer's movement and achieve remarkable changes in attitudes: no longer mindless empty shells, we were being listened to and included.

Throughout much of this book you will read references to these wonderful colleagues in DASNI. I have given several talks over the years about the impact that this group of 'heroes' has made. As Margaret Mead, the anthropologist, is thought to have said: 'Never doubt that a small group of thoughtful, committed citizens can change the world.' Since then, many of us have slowed down over the years, so that our collective voice was weakening. But then in 2014 – 'on the shoulders of these giants' – the Dementia Alliance International (DAI – www. dementiaallianceinternational.org) was established. Communications and social media have come a long way since 2001, and DAI is able to hold regular café-style webinars, publish newsletters and lobby for change. It not only encourages people with dementia but also forms a powerful collective voice for the inclusion of and participation by people with dementia in the global effort to listen to the experts on the lived experience of dementia, and to improve the care of people with dementia.

For me it has been a remarkable journey, to see such change, such progress and so many positive outcomes. But there is still much to do. I have lasted 20 years since my diagnosis. I'm still here, still speaking out, still doing my best to let people know what it is like to have dementia and what you can do to help. However, there has been a steady decline in my thinking and speaking ability and the consistency of my behaviour over that time, which is increasingly affecting my daily life. I cope as best I can, with my dear husband Paul's support, and I will continue my efforts for as long as possible.

Of course, I hope that I will last long enough to see a cure for the form of dementia that I have, but I am very much aware that dementia is the result of more than 100 different diseases, each causing increasing damage to the brain.

How many cures will there need to be? Even if a cure or cures are found, we will still need to strive to improve the care of people with dementia. Just as for cancer, we need to ensure we strive for the best possible care during diagnosis and treatment.

I look forward to the day when all forms of dementia become treatable conditions and we receive the best possible care and support during any treatment and recovery, but this, I fear, will be a long way off. In the meantime, I will do my best to shine and surprise, despite my many limitations.

My husband, Paul, wanted to put together an edited selection of my many talks over the years, before I died! He felt it would be important to capture much of my thinking and to reach out to a wider audience than just those who had listened to some of my talks or viewed them in video clips or on my website. Paul thought it would be a way to encourage so many more people with dementia, their families and care workers. This was the germ of an idea that resulted in this collection of talks. I needed his help with the footnotes and the many copyediting issues that arose during the preparation of the book, including some misquotes, which have been corrected or acknowledged.

These talks have been reproduced much in the form that they were given, and cover two decades. Therefore, you will see that some terminology seems outdated, even obsolete. For example, we now talk of dementia being a condition rather than an illness or disease. Also I was on a couple of earlier forms of anti-dementia medication (as well as some complementary medication, which later research showed to be less effective).

My talks chart years of change, but there is still much to be done. I hope new generations of leaders, care workers and managers will be encouraged to do all they can to help improve the encouragement, care and support given to people with dementia. I am delighted at the attention now being given to dementia and the leadership that has been shown in establishing the G7 World Dementia Council. I'll do my best to stay around and see the outcomes from this global endeavour!

Christine Bryden
Brisbane
February 2015

1

Dementia diagnosis – 'pointing the bone'

Christine Bryden and Morris Friedell

Dementia Advocacy and Support Network International (DASNI)

March 2001[1]

Christine   I'm Christine Bryden. I was diagnosed in 1995 with Alzheimer's; then, in 1998, this was revised to fronto-temporal dementia. I wrote a book about my struggles, called *Who will I be when I die?*[2] Last year I met over the internet my co-presenter, Morris Friedell, who has Alzheimer's. He introduced me to a great support group for people with memory loss.

This group set up the Dementia Advocacy and Support Network International (DASNI) in September 2000. This is a non-profit organization set up by and for people diagnosed with dementia, who work together to improve our quality of life. It is a great privilege to give this keynote address on behalf of our colleagues in DASNI, from the US, Canada, Australia and the UK.

Our talk argues that the trauma of diagnosis changes the person and their family, because they respond as if the Aboriginal sorcerer had pointed the bone at the victim, and he or she is doomed to die. We challenge the view of inevitable decline and highlight some typical dysfunctional responses to the 'pointing-bone' of diagnosis.

---

1   Plenary presentation to the Alzheimer's Australia 9th National Conference, Canberra, March 2001, drafted and presented with Professor Morris Friedell, whom Christine had met over the internet in collaborating in dementia advocacy by people with dementia.

2   Christine Bryden (2012) *Who will I be when I die?* London: Jessica Kingsley Publishers (first published 1998).

What's happened since speaking to National Conference Sept '99?

Meeting Morris – a fellow flying turtle in cyberspace!

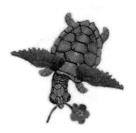

Before we start our talk – a quick update. I gave a talk at the last National Conference in 1999 about my personal experience of living positively with dementia. There was no one else with dementia at that conference in Perth, so I'm delighted that many of my colleagues with memory loss – the real experts on many of the things we are talking about – are here today.

Since then I have completed a graduate diploma, specializing in counselling of people with dementia, and continued to give talks and write articles on what it is like to have dementia. Although my brain continues to disappear, I keep trying new things and have a positive outlook.

Last year I joined an email support group for people with dementia, and met many others like me, who wanted to share and encourage each other. My new friends are in the US and Canada, but in many ways are closer to me than the 'normals' I meet each day.

Morris is one of these new friends, a fellow flying turtle – which is the DASNI logo. Turtle-like in our cognition, the wings signify angels helping us rise to the heights of our abilities, drawing on our emotional sensitivity and spirituality.

This paper represents our shared thinking on the issue of dementia, and what the experience of diagnosis means to us and our family.

Dementia...far more than just brain damage

Surely we are more than simply a mass of brain tissue – we have emotions, experiences and a place in a social world.

Our psychic resources affect how we cope with:

▸ brain damage and
▸ the trauma of diagnosis.

Morris and I are far more than simply diseased brains. We each have a unique personality with emotions, experiences and a place in a social world. We have drawn on our own psychic resources to cope with our brain damage and the difficulties we are experiencing in our daily lives. Most importantly, we needed these resources at the moment of diagnosis, which was a terrible trauma.

At first I know I reacted to this trauma by believing the lie of dementia – that I would decline and there was no hope. My family believed this too, and became very caring – but far too caring – and smothered me. They took the identity of 'carer'. But in the end I was able to cast this lie aside and challenge accepted wisdom.

Morris had a similar traumatic experience and reacted by focusing on how to die with dignity just before the end stage. His family found it hard to believe anything was wrong, adopting the identity of 'denier'. They did not help him face his demons. But, like me, he has been able to draw on his psychic resources and now is leading our thinking on rehabilitation for dementia.

Half empty or half full?

We have cast aside the cloudy half-empty glass of dementia's past.

Like our friend Dan on DANSI:

> 'We raise up our crystal-clear half-full mug…with the help of doctors, friends and God we will not let dementia become the centre of our life.'

We rejected the dementia script: 'Don't push yourself, better safe than sorry.' We fought off depression, demoralization, to live for today and tomorrow with dignity and cheerfulness. Like our friend Dan on DASNI, 'we raise up our crystal-clear half-full mug' of living positively with dementia.

The cloudy half-empty glass of dementia's past developed in the framework of diagnosis only after years of memory loss and confusion, without the assistance of sophisticated scanning techniques to show up the earlier signs of brain damage.

In this cloudy past there were no anti-dementia drugs to keep us functioning at our current levels for as long as possible. And there were no support groups – in the flesh or in cyberspace – in which we could encourage each other to live positively with dementia.

Now our doctors can prescribe anti-dementia drugs after an earlier diagnosis, so we can function at a far higher level than ever thought possible before. We have access to support networks and find others like ourselves who can laugh over our frailties, share our despair and encourage each other with helpful tips.

'For Thou art with me'

Our spirituality helps us maintain:

- ▸ personhood and
- ▸ emotional sensitivity.

It can flourish as cognition fades to give us:

- ▸ identity and
- ▸ meaning as a transcendent being.

Importantly, in the face of declining cognition and increasing emotional sensitivity, our spirituality can flourish as an important source of identity – of personhood.

Our self, which feels at risk through the dreaded decline of dementia, can be given meaning as a transcendent being. Our sense of self is shattered and can be restored in a relationship with God, in which our emotional sensitivity is affirmed. Often our worldly relationships have been terribly altered by the diagnosis – we have become a victim and our family may find a new identity as carer or denier.

Throughout all of this our spirituality can remain our mainstay. For Morris as a Jew and for me as a Christian, it has been an important source of hope and meaning in our lives. Yea, though I walk through the valley of the shadow of death, I will fear no evil. For Thou art with me.

The rumblings of catastrophe

When our world begins to fall apart…

our social context is critical in how we deal with:

▸ our cognitive decline and

▸ the toxic power of the 'bone-pointing' moment of diagnosis.

Often the first signs of our dementia are seen at times of stress, and we withdraw from challenging situations as a defence against failure. Our world begins to fall apart as we sense the rumblings of catastrophe.

We increasingly use avoidance, and allow others in our social context – usually our family – to take over our functioning, often to the stage where we 'forget' how to do it ourselves. 'Use it or lose it' is painfully true for us, and we risk losing everything by our learned helplessness.

And then we face the toxic power of the 'pointing-bone' of diagnosis, when it seems as if our world has come to an end. We experience a defeat of spirit and of hope. We feel extreme fear of further loss, and dread what the future holds.

Morris joined the Hemlock Society[3] in reaction to this existential fear. I did not know what function I would lose next, and each mistake became a sign of irreversible decline. I withdrew into depression, masked by apparent contentment.

---

3   The Hemlock Society USA was a national right-to-die organization founded in 1980. In 2004 it merged with another group to form Compassion and Choices.

NOTHING ABOUT US, WITHOUT US!

'Pointing the bone'

As our friend Carole on DASNI said:

'One moment you are a vital intimate partner in your relationships, the next you are merely a custodial obligation like a pet, a mortgage or yesterday's laundry…

…and expected to withdraw from the world's stage, assigned only the smallest walk-on parts.'

As our friend Carole on DASNI said, 'the day before our diagnosis, we each could be vital and intimate partners in our personal relationships. The day after we had become a liability, like a pet, a mortgage or yesterday's laundry.'

We were no longer respected. Morris was a sociology professor; I was a senior public servant. Overnight each of us had become simply another case of dementia. We were expected to withdraw from the world's stage and be assigned only the smallest walk-on parts. For me, it seemed as if from then on I would only ever be allowed to function with my 'carer' in attendance.

How come so much had changed overnight?

How our family reacts can be critical in helping us cope

If it accepts the diagnosis, tells us to stop, adopts the identity of 'carer':

- ‣ we usually give up and
- ‣ exhibit learned helplessness.

It's our primitive defence against fear or failure: we let the carer take over.

How our family reacts can be critical in helping us cope, particularly at that moment of diagnosis. There are two dysfunctional ways in which our families can react: to adopt the role of 'carer' or 'denier'. There is a middle way, but so often one of these reactions is what occurs, at least at the first shock of diagnosis.

My home and church family initially adopted the identity of 'carer'. They did things for me and expected little of me. I responded by learned helplessness. I stopped answering the phone, found reading difficult and writing impossible. I gave up driving. It was all too hard.

It was my defence against failure, against humiliation. Against further confirmation that I was losing it. You see, each time I failed at something, I thought I would never be able to do that thing again. I believed it was a sign of having lost yet another function for good. I did not keep trying.

I believed the lie of dementia.

How our family reacts can be critical in helping us cope

If it rejects the diagnosis, runs away, adopts the role of 'denier', we cover up, struggling for normalcy.

It's our way of accepting the message: dementia is too dreadful to be dealt with.

Morris My family denied I had a problem. That was their defence against feelings of grief and anger. The implicit message was that dementia was far too dreadful to deal with constructively. In mitigation, my clinical symptoms did not look representative of any dementia, but like an exacerbation of my long-standing non-verbal learning disorder.

Often persons with a pre-existing neurological or psychiatric condition have particular problems with family denial. They say, 'He's always been that way.'

Or indeed the family may have a history of dysfunction. My children's mother frequently threatened suicide or homicide when they were small, but did not make serious efforts to act on these threats. This probably was in the background of their reaction.

The denial pushed me to maintain a facade of normalcy, which then tended to increase the denial. And occasionally I'd get hysterical out of desperation or frustration, which made my problem look psychiatric rather than neurological. Thank God for a therapist familiar with brain damage, for a few old friends and for internet buddies.

Let's show you our 'bones'

Our brain scans are our 'pointing-bones'…and made us into victims.

Morris's PET scan report, August 1998

> Conclusion: This study is consistent with an early Alzheimer's disease pattern.

At this point it is important to assert to you that we truly are persons with brain damage – persons with dementia. Our brain scans are our 'pointing-bones'.

I have my report from a PET[4] scan taken at the University of California Los Angeles Nuclear Medicine Clinic, in August 1998.

Findings: There is mild hypometabolism seen throughout the cortical structures. The presence of mild widening of the interfissural space, intercaudate space, and interthalami space, suggest evidence of mild atrophy. Additional superimposed mild hypometabolism is seen over the right temporal lobe and bilateral parietal lobes.

Conclusion: This study is consistent with an early Alzheimer's disease pattern.

---

4 A positron emission tomography (PET) scan uses a radioactive trace substance to look at how the body (in this case the brain) functions.

NOTHING ABOUT US, WITHOUT US!

Christine's PET scan report, July 1998

Conclusion: … The findings are consistent with a fronto-temporal dementia…

The report of Christine's scan, taken in July 1998 at the Royal Prince Alfred Hospital in Sydney, says:

There has been definite but slight progression in the degree of cerebral hypometabolism and atrophy, which is most marked in the mid to superior frontal lobes.

The interhemispheric fissure is much wider than three years ago and is associated with a more marked reduction in metabolism in the mesial frontal cortex, particularly in the region of the cingulate gyrus.

There is relative sparing of the orbito-frontal cortex and the lateral frontal cortex, which is also reflected in the relative preservation of metabolism in the striatum and thalami.

There is also hypometabolism of both temporal lobes with a suggestion of temporal lobe atrophy bilaterally. All the changes are more marked on the right.

Conclusion: There is mild but definite progression since the scan three years ago. The findings are consistent with a front-temporal dementia rather than the pattern seen with dementia of the Alzheimer type.

There is life after diagnosis

Not giving up, nor covering up. Although our lives changed forever, we challenge you with our level of functioning.

But are we really that exceptional?

Our brain scans symbolize the moment of diagnosis, when our lives changed forever. By giving this talk and functioning in this context, we are challenging the view that the person with dementia must lack insight, ability or judgement.

We are not giving up, nor are we covering up. Although we retain our ability to do intellectual work and present it in public using carefully prepared notes, we are open about our diseases that have drastically changed our lifestyles.

For example, I live near beautiful mountains but cannot enjoy hiking in them because my impaired parietal lobes quickly become fatigued by visual processing. I have five beautiful grandchildren, but I can hardly baby-sit for them because my impaired frontal lobes make my judgement unreliable in stressful situations.

You may be tempted to think that we are somehow misdiagnosed, or the disease hasn't hit us, or that our ability to function here is so exceptional that it is irrelevant to other persons with dementia.

But what if...?

...we were young persons with brain damage after a car accident...and we were given rehabilitation and a vital hope of future possibilities?

...we people with dementia were no longer assigned to a 'hospice in slow motion'?

But what if we were young persons who had suffered head impact in a motor accident and had analogous diffuse brain damage? And suppose we had rich and loving parents who sent us to top-notch rehabilitation programs and nourished us with vital hope that we could recover rich and productive lives?

Our success then would not be so strange. Comparatively, all that is given to persons with dementia is 'hospice in slow motion'. We reject this. There is life after a diagnosis of dementia, for both ourselves and our families.

There is no need for the roles of carer, denier or victim.

What's the toxic lie of dementia?

We're biologically inferior because of our abnormal brains.

But didn't we win the war! People are no longer judged on the basis of concepts of biological inferiority.

God created us to love and serve him, not to be emotionally normal.

Our brain scans are abnormal, but what does this really mean? We both have frontal lobe damage. Statistical probabilities are that we are childish, apathetic, irritable and impulsive. The biological facts severely challenge us, but we are unique individuals. There is much about the brain – and about the consciousness somehow connected with it – that remains a mystery.

The toxic lie is that our abnormal brains make us biologically inferior. Haven't I heard about 'biological inferiority' somewhere before? The Nazis…the Holocaust… We won World War II, didn't we? Didn't our fathers fight for a world where persons are no longer judged by some concept of biological inferiority?

The Amnesty International 2001 calendar has a beautiful message from survivors of imprisonment and torture: 'Let no one tell you that your hands are bound!'

Let no one tell you that because your frontal lobes are damaged and you have tendencies to be childish or apathetic, you must be enslaved by these tendencies. In religious terms, we could say God created us to love and serve him, not to be emotionally normal.

Exorcism

No shame, no pretence, nor withdrawal.

Living a contradiction – an exorcism – to the toxic lie of dementia, countering the 'pointing-bone' of diagnosis.

To face and surmount challenges, affirming our courage and dignity.

We believe there's no true shame in being mentally disabled – the shame would be in covering up as if there weren't more important things in the world than normalcy. Neither pretence at normalcy nor withdrawal into learned helplessness is the way to respond to the pointing-bone.

- What if we retain neuroplasticity, the capacity to learn?
- What if we could throw off the role of victim?
- What if we could stop pretending at normalcy and address the challenge of dementia?

We need to live a contradiction to the toxic lie of dementia – to live an exorcism, as it were, countering the curse of the pointing-bone of diagnosis. We can be guided to simple therapeutic behaviours in which failure is unlikely and through which we can start to recover our shattered sense of competence.

We can discover ways of participating in life through giving and caring which restore our sense of value and meaning. Thus strengthened, we find that again we can face and surmount challenges, and affirm our courage and dignity.

Let's open the door…

…to a wider world of possibilities.

…to a new identity as survivor, no longer in our prison of helpless victim or hopeless pretender.

We can be encouraged to open the door to a wider world of possibilities.

The theme of our discussion sessions for people with dementia this week has been 'Education in possibility'. The concept is to find new horizons despite our limitations.

No longer enclosed in the prison of helpless victim or hopeless pretender, we can find a new identity as survivor. Our family is released from a role as denier or carer, and can walk alongside us as we rediscover who we can be – living positively with dementia. No longer frozen by a denier or smothered by a carer, we discover a survivor mission.

NOTHING ABOUT US, WITHOUT US!

Our survivor mission

Like Martin Luther King, we know what it feels like to suffer from a 'degenerating sense of nobodiness'.

We in DASNI aspire to be a great people – persons with dementia – 'who injected new meaning and dignity into the veins of civilization'.

We know what it feels like to have the 'degenerating sense of nobodiness' that oppressed Martin Luther King's fellow black Americans. Yet we have also been in the world of normalcy, where you 'temporarily able-brained' persons live.

It's as if we are bilingual or bicultural. Exiled from our past lifestyle, we have lots of time to deeply and creatively relate. And we are conscious of the preciousness of our brief sojourn on earth. Having survived trauma, we know our strength. Our cognition may be fading, but we can draw on powerful resources – our emotions and our spirituality – to relate to you.

It is you who must stretch yourselves to empathize with us, and, having been where you are, we can reach out across the divide to touch you in a new way.

We in DASNI are inspired by Martin Luther King's formulation of his people's survivor mission:

> If you will protest courageously and yet with dignity and Christian love, when the history books are written in future generations, the historians will have to pause and say: there lived a great people – a black people – who injected new meaning and dignity into the veins of civilization.[5]

We in DASNI also aspire to be such a people – another great people: persons with dementia.

5   This was part of a speech King made during the bus boycott in Montgomery, Alabama on 5 December 1955. It was cited by Gunnar Jahn, chairman of the Nobel Committee on 10 December 1964 (www. nobelprize.org/nobel_prizes/peace/laureates/1964/press.html).

Our vision

The 'D' word has lost its toxic power to create deniers, carers and victims.

Our families walk alongside us as we build a new life in a world that:

- ▸ focuses on relationships rather than cognition and
- ▸ regards emotional and spiritual healing
  more highly than physical healing.

Christine So what is our vision for the new millennium? We remember when cancer was the dreaded 'C word'. We are inspired by cancer survivors, and we look forward to a new future in which the 'D word' – or that 'A word' of Alzheimer's – has lost its toxic power to create deniers, carers and victims.

In this brave new world, people with cognitive difficulties seek out diagnosis as early as possible, so that they can be prescribed anti-dementia medication and retain function at the highest possible level for as long as possible.

I have been on these medications for nearly six years now. I cannot function without them, and would have lost a lot of function had I had a later diagnosis or not been prescribed them immediately.

Our vision is a world which has moved away from hyper-cognition to a focus on relationships – between people, with the land, and with God – when the stigma of dementia will be a thing of the past.

We will walk alongside our families to find a new identity that is not cast by any role held before diagnosis, nor cast by any pretence at normalcy or withdrawal into helplessness. This will take courage, to build a new life and to achieve emotional and spiritual healing.

A new paradigm

We have a dream of future possibilities where there is dementia survival with dignity.

Let's be companions 'together on a journey' towards transforming our culture to one honouring humankind as created in the divine image.

We have a dream of future possibilities. Our resources lie in self-reflection, courage, imagination and prayer. We don't want to be blind to our potential. It's harder for us – but not impossible. We want you to help us realize our dream, and want Alzheimer's associations around the world to aspire to a new paradigm of dementia survival with dignity.

As dementia survivors, we know both the world of 'normals' and that of dementia intimately, and we have weathered an extraordinary transition.

By making this presentation, we are claiming our full participation in cultural life and making a stand for all people with cognitive limitations. Morris and I are in solidarity as Christian and Jew, as persons with Alzheimer's and fronto-temporal dementia, as Australian and American.

We seek to work towards transforming our culture to one honouring human dignity – or humankind as created in the divine image. Let's be companions together on this journey towards dementia survival with dignity.

2

Diagnosis, drugs and determination

Christine Bryden

Dementia Advocacy and Support Network International (DASNI)

October 2001[1]

My name is Christine Bryden, and I have fronto-temporal dementia. I think I am the first person with dementia to give a plenary address at Alzheimer's Disease International and I am sure there will be many others in the years to come.

I am a member of the Board of the Dementia Advocacy and Support Network International (or DASNI), which is an organization set up by and for people with dementia. We have around 130 members around the world.

At this conference we are being well represented, including running a booth, a workshop on co-dependency and discussion sessions for people with dementia. This is a world first and I commend ADI and the New Zealand organizing committee for being open to our participation and willing to take the risk of including us.

You have heard about dementia from a professional perspective, about medication and about research. I'd like to introduce a different perspective: that of the consumer, the client, of these services – the person who is being diagnosed with dementia.

---

1   Plenary presentation to the Alzheimer's Disease International (ADI) 17th Biennial Conference, Christchurch, October 2001. Christine was the first person with dementia to be invited to address ADI.

From diagnosis to death

What does this journey start?

A kaleidoscope of problems:

- something's not quite right
- irritability, tiredness, stress
- gaps in memory.

Life's an inside struggle and an uphill battle.

'It feels like I am clinging to a precipice with my fingernails.'

We people with dementia, together with our families, are on a journey from diagnosis to death. Dementia is now a major health problem, not merely one of ageing and aged care, and is set to become the major disabling disease in women in Australia over the next five to ten years This perspective can affect the service you might provide to us, for we will have needs maybe long before we begin to exhibit what you might call challenging behaviour.

Our journey begins with a struggle with daily life, of tiredness, irritability, stress, a feeling that not all is well. There may well be gaps in our memory, but that is not always the first sign we feel.

It's more like a kaleidoscope of small problems, of not quite being ourselves. We don't do everything we used to do; it all seems so much trouble. It's what you on the outside of our inside struggle might call apathy. But it's not lack of interest, but a lack of energy.

In stressful situations we cope very poorly, as we have so few additional resources to muster under such a strain. Ordinary life takes up all we have. As I said in my book *Who will I be when I die?*[2] 'It feels like I am clinging to a precipice with my fingernails. It takes all my effort to stay where I am.'

---

2   Christine Bryden (2012) *Who will I be when I die?* London: Jessica Kingsley Publishers (first published 1998).

NOTHING ABOUT US, WITHOUT US!

Tests, tension, apprehension

Subjecting ourselves to the medical process:

‣ the insult of MMSE

‣ scary scans and other tests

‣ impersonal medical reports.

The agony of waiting, wondering…let it be something that can be treated and cured, I don't want to lose my very self.

The first step along our journey is one of laying ourselves open to the medical profession, of a series of tests, of tension and of apprehension. This is a traumatic time for us and our families.

There is the insult of the MMSE,[3] or, if we are lucky, full neuro-psychological testing, when we find out that we cannot put a series of pictures together, or blocks, or remember a shopping list. We feel like failures.

We face a battery of impersonal medical reports, with one-line summaries, saying, 'Generalized atrophy. No other abnormality. Thank you for referring this patient' (from my first CT scan). The brain scans can be very scary, lying claustrophobically inside what feels like a torpedo tube, outside which roadwork is going on, or a loud techno party raging. One of the two.

During all these tests there is the agony of waiting, wondering and desperately hoping that it will be something that can be treated and cured. But at the same time we feel safe: something is being done about the problems we have felt.

---

3   The Mini Mental State Examination (MMSE) is a 30-point questionnaire used to measure cognitive impairment.

That moment of diagnosis…

…is etched in our memories, like the day when President Kennedy died.

Trauma, disbelief or relief.

Waving the distress flag as our ship of life sinks, we feel helpless, powerless, and we've lost our identity.

It may have been months or even years before we have got to this moment of testing. Our GPs may fail to recognize the signs of dementia, particularly in younger people, or dismiss our difficulties as simply a case of 'getting old'. Both we and our families have struggled to get to this point, but we wait in fearful apprehension.

Finally, after the tension of tests, there is the moment of diagnosis. For many of us it is etched in our memories, like the day President Kennedy died. The experience can be one of extreme trauma, or of disbelief, or even relief (at last there is acknowledgment of our difficulties). Often there is a lack of information, of hope and of compassion at this critical moment for us.

The diagnosis is a turning point, at which we must face the awful awareness of what lies ahead in terms of possible further losses. We feel like waving a flag of distress, as our ship of life sinks. We are experiencing a continuing threat to self, and feelings of helplessness and powerlessness. Our identity that we had prior to diagnosis is destroyed. All these experiences are like those that lead to chronic trauma.

Becoming a labelled person

A label 'dementia' is attached and we become depersonalized.

It feels like a big stop sign has just been placed on our life's path.

The stigma of dementia has joined us on our journey, which we and our family face together with fear and uncertainty.

Not only must we cope with this internal turmoil, but now we have become a labelled person. We are yet another case of Alzheimer's or dementia. Our inner fear at loss of self, of identity, is exacerbated by this outer stripping away of who we once were.

It feels like a big stop sign has just been placed on our life's path, and we cannot see beyond to any new future – only a journey further into dementia. This journey seems full of more stop signs – of stopping work, stopping driving, stopping golf, stopping looking after grandchildren.

Our brand-new label of dementia is like the Yellow Star of the Jew of the ghetto; we have the stigma of 'being demented'. We are watched carefully for odd behaviour, we are not able to be trusted, we are thought to lack insight, our input is not taken seriously, and we are expected to start wandering, getting lost and exhibiting challenging behaviour.

Rachel Remen says that 'diagnosis is simply another form of judgement'.[4] It is a critical step on our journey, to a future of stop signs which we and our family face together with fear and uncertainty.

---

4   Rachel Remen (1998) *Kitchen Table Wisdom*. Australia: Pan Macmillan, p.233.

Targeted by stigma...blindfolded by fear

Our lives become limited by stigma, almost as if a target was painted on our forehead.

We retreat in shame, blindfolded to our own potential.

Our inner world is in turmoil as we suffer anticipatory grief at loss of self and of others.

Diagnosis has changed our world forever. Our lives become limited by the stigma we face in the world around us. It's like we have a target painted on our foreheads shouting out 'dementing' for all the world to see. People become awkward in our presence, are unsure of our behaviour, and our world becomes circumscribed by the stigma of our illness.

We want to retreat in shame, and do not want to 'come out' and tell people the diagnosis. It's not surprising that some of us react by denying anything is wrong, and our families do too. Better to pretend at normalcy than to face up to the challenge of dementia.

If we do believe the lie of dementia – that we can't learn new things, remember reliably or find our way around – we are blindfolded to our own potential. We withdraw into helplessness and let our families take over.

Our inner world is in turmoil as we suffer anticipatory grief at loss of self. We may become overwhelmed by feelings of anxiety, anger, sadness, fatigue, shock, helplessness and numbness as we try to come to terms with losing ourselves as well as others.

But is that diagnosis right?

Often we're labelled Alzheimer's:

- ▸ But what about fronto-temporal dementia (FTD), vascular dementia, Lewy Body dementia?
- ▸ What about our access to anti-dementia medication?

But is that devastating diagnosis right? So often we are given the label 'Alzheimer's', but what about fronto-temporal dementia (FTD), vascular dementia, Lewy Body dementia? Still devastating, but you may need to offer other types of treatment. The current prevalence of Alzheimer's may be incorrect, because autopsy checks show 40–60 per cent of cases were another type of dementia. FTD probably accounts for 20 per cent of cases of degenerative dementia. It is inherited in around 40 per cent of cases – far higher than in Alzheimer's. It took three years for my original diagnosis of Alzheimer's to be revised to FTD and only now must I deal with this issue.

Anti-dementia drug research is on groups of people with Alzheimer's, because that is what many of us are told we have at first. The drugs are trialled and have good effect, but how many people in that research cohort actually had some other form of dementia? Tragically, the drugs may be denied to people with other forms of dementia, because the results supposedly only apply to Alzheimer's. This may only be around 50–60 per cent of cases of dementia, of those in the research group. What about the rest of us, who could also benefit?

'When I have fears that I may cease to be'

Give us information about dementia; don't assume we lack insight.

What about counselling and support groups?

Help us to 'bear witness to the uniquely human potential…to transform a personal tragedy into a triumph'.

Like the poet John Keats, expressing a fear of death, we can say of diagnosis that this is a time 'When I have fears that I may cease to be'. If we are labelled, we are susceptible to fear. Like Viktor Frankl, help us 'to bear witness to the uniquely human potential…which is to transform a personal tragedy into a triumph, to turn one's predicament into a human achievement'.[5]

What do you tell us at this critical time of diagnosis? 'It's best not to let her know.' 'He doesn't really understand.' 'Go home and enjoy the rest of your life.' The assumption is that nothing can be done, so why bother? But we want to get our life in order, to think about family relationships, our legal and financial affairs. Give us information about dementia. Don't assume we lack insight, for we might simply be in denial – a perfectly normal response to the shock of diagnosis. What about counselling and support groups? This could help us work through our grief over losing our self, and our family and friends, during the course of the disease. Symptoms of dementia may be exacerbated by the grief reaction, as we experience anxiety, anger, sadness, fatigue, shock, helplessness and numbness.

---

5   Viktor E. Frankl (1985) *Man's Search for Meaning*. New York: Washington Square Press, p.135.

NOTHING ABOUT US, WITHOUT US!

Remember: treatment delayed is treatment denied

DO NOT DELAY!

Give us anti-dementia medication at the moment of diagnosis to slow further decline.

Advise us to consider complementary medication.

We need any resources you can give us at that critical turning point of diagnosis, to help us retain cognitive skills to work through our issues, as a springboard to greater spiritual and emotional strength.

The most important thing to do at the moment of diagnosis is to give us anti-dementia drugs to slow further decline. Do not delay! Remember: treatment delayed is treatment denied.

These drugs – cholinesterase inhibitors – act to inhibit the breakdown of a chemical messenger in our brain, so helping what remains to work better. They seem to keep us where we are, not recapture what we have lost, so it is important to start them as early as possible. Not only do they help our cognitive function, they also help with our behaviour and general function.

Complementary medicines are also important. Check with your doctor which ones may help.

I have been taking a form of anti-dementia medication since 1995, and also I like to keep abreast of the latest in research on complementary medications, in case they might also help me.

What the medications do for us

Without them, it's a fog.

They give our life back and give us the key to a new future.

But we still ebb and flow like a parallel universe of untreated and treated dementia.

Without the medications, it's like thinking in fog and walking through treacle. The tablets (or patches) give our life back and give us the key to a new future. We can think more clearly, feel less tired and be more in control of our lives and our behaviour.

But we still ebb and flow like a parallel universe of untreated and treated dementia. We have our good days and our bad days. As my friend Morris has said, there are 'windows of clarity' which we must take advantage of.

Unpredictably, we can feel exhausted, confused, muddle-headed. Life seems too difficult and we retreat. We may even experience what you call a catastrophic reaction when life becomes too much to deal with. But remember, dementia is an abnormal situation. As Viktor Frankl has said: 'An abnormal reaction to an abnormal situation is normal behaviour.'[6]

But without anti-dementia medication or complementary medicines, this abnormal behaviour is how it would be all the time.

---

6   Viktor E. Frankl (1985) *Man's Search for Meaning*. New York: Washington Square Press, p.38.

Moving from being a victim to becoming a survivor

The challenge is to draw on our psychic resources, personality and biography to step across that yawning chasm of fear that opened up at that moment of diagnosis.

By our attitude, we can create a new image of who we are becoming and find meaning in our lives.

After diagnosis and medication comes determination. We who have experienced the trauma of a diagnosis of dementia, and are relatively stable on medication, now must try to move from being a victim to becoming a survivor.

The challenge is to draw on our psychic resources to step across that yawning chasm of fear that opened up at the moment of diagnosis. How can we live in a world of hope, alternatives, growth and possibility when dementia threatens our sense of self?

We need to create a new image of who we are and who we are becoming. How we do this depends very much on our personality, our life story, our health, our spirituality and our social environment. We can choose the attitude we have, and, like Frankl, look for meaning in our lives through the attitude we take towards unavoidable suffering.

We need to make sure we do not retreat into helplessness and let you take over our functioning, nor try to act as if we are normal and then become stressed at how difficult this is.

'It is the artist's task to find out how much music you can still make with what you have left'

Discovering new talents, focusing on relationships, emotions, spirituality.

Assigning cognition a secondary place, being content with life in the slow lane we have 'time to prepare for a new future' and find peace.

Like Itzhak Perlman, the violinist who needs crutches to get on stage, we people with dementia have a vital task on our journey with dementia: 'It is the artist's task to find out how much music you can still make with what you have left.'[7] Like him, we must often struggle to cope, to create, to dazzle, despite our limitations.

We can discover new talents, focusing on relationships, emotions, spirituality, rather than on cognition. By assigning cognition a secondary place, being content with our new life in the slow lane, we can enhance these other aspects of our personality.

Many of us have learned how to communicate over the internet, finding great joy in encouraging each other and deep support in sharing with others. We have made new friends in our support groups and have become much more attuned to our emotions than ever before.

Many of us can identify with Basil Hume, when he was diagnosed with cancer: 'I have received two wonderful graces. First the time to prepare for a new future. Secondly, I find myself – uncharacteristically – calm and at peace.'[8]

---

7   These words are attributed to Perlman after he supposedly finished a concert with a violin with three strings after one string broke. The story was published in the *Houston Chronicle* on 10 February 2001 but it seems there may be no truth in it. The words are nevertheless very powerful.

8   These words of Basil Hume, English cardinal from the 1970s to the 1990s, are cited in the section on 'Dying' in *The Oxford Dictionary of Thematic Quotations* (Susan Ratcliffe (ed.) 2000, Oxford University Press).

'Transforming the patterns of our life is always done in our heart'

We need to find out what we can celebrate on this journey with dementia.

The fleas in Ravensbrück kept away the guards for Betsie Ten Boom.

'Life is 10 per cent what actually happens to us, and 90 per cent how we react to it.'

In *A Path with Heart*, Jack Kornfield says we can change our inner attitude, and this is enough to transform our life. We can choose how we will react to our new life in the slow lane, realizing that 'transforming the patterns of our life is always done in our heart'.[9]

So our first step is to find out what we can celebrate. We choose to find joy in being sensitive in our relationships, in being open to our spirituality, and finding positive aspects of living in the slow lane.

For me, dementia meant retiring from work and being able to pick up my daughters after school in the light, rather than race to see them in the dark after a long day at work.

For Betsie Ten Boom in the concentration camp horror of Ravensbrück, the fleas were a godsend, keeping away the guards.

As Charles Swindoll has said, life is 10 per cent what actually happens to us, and 90 per cent how we react to it.[10]

It is through finding meaning
in life, even in dementia,
that we can create a new
sense of becoming and
overcome fear of loss.

---

9   Kornfield, J. (1993) *A Path with Heart*. Random House, Kindle edition, p.276.
10   Charles Swindoll is a pastor, author, educator and radio preacher.

What you can't feel, you can't heal

We're on a path to healing through feeling.

Casting aside the lie of dementia, we can create a new future.

Bridging the gap between our world and yours, we help you understand us and our needs.

What you can't feel, you can't heal. Rachel Remen says that the part that feels joy is the same that feels suffering. By working through our fear, we can begin to feel joy. We are on a path to healing, through feeling and acknowledging our fear, anxiety and the ebbs and flow of confusion. By casting aside the lie of dementia, we can work towards creating a new future. We need to realize that our passage through diagnosis, medication – and now through to determination – will be a struggle of feeling to achieve healing. Most importantly, on this journey, we can come to realize that we are uniquely qualified to reach out to you, our families and friends walking alongside us on this journey with dementia.

We have been where you are, in the world of normals, and know what that feels like intimately. But you have no idea what it feels like for us. We are bicultural, bilingual, speaking and knowing the language and mores of normality as well as dementia. So we can bridge the gap between the world of normality and the world of dementia, and help you to understand us and our needs.

A fine balance…

…between pretending at normalcy and withdrawing into helplessness.

What is normal in this abnormal disease?

Reclaiming my life with realism and humour, with you alongside me as a partner in my endeavour.

In reaching out to you, we must maintain a fine balance between pretending at normalcy and withdrawing into helplessness. What is normal in this abnormal disease? We can be tempted to maintain a cheerful facade and deny anything is wrong. You may either go along with this and deny dementia or assume we lack insight and take over our lives.

We cannot win. If we both pretend at normalcy, remember that increasing energy is required to maintain the self, so less is available for you and for coping with stress. We may show a catastrophic reaction to what may seem to you to be a simple challenge.

If you take over our life, then it is so easy for us to withdraw into helplessness. Life is so hard anyway, and you can make it so much easier for us. But in so doing, we who need constant repeating of actions and thoughts to keep remembering lose functions daily. The challenge for me is to reclaim my life with realism and humour, with you alongside me as a partner in this endeavour.

Getting back into the driving seat of life!

Confronting the fear of a living death, drawing on our inner resources.

Finding the pearl hidden within us.

Working together to build a new future, by sharing, supporting and encouraging.

Determination is about getting back into the driving seat of life. We are confronting the fear of a living death, drawing on our inner resources. We can overcome our feelings of inertia, of exhaustion, as we face this journey of dementia with courage.

We need to find the pearl hidden within us. Like a pearl formed through the irritation of a grain of sand within an oyster, our pearl has formed through the challenge of living with dementia.

Finding this pearl within is the key to transforming the patterns of our life and creating a new future of life in the slow lane.

We can work together as people with dementia in discussion groups, such as happened at the Alzheimer's Australia National Conference 2001 and is happening at this ADI Conference, or in support groups in our home countries, or as part of an internet-based support network. As a group of people who share the same world, the world of living with dementia, we can find our hidden pearls, working together to build a new future, by sharing, supporting and encouraging each other.

Horizons of hope

Liberation from internalizing the oppressor of dementia.

'As we are liberated from our own fear, our presence automatically liberates others.'

We seek a new paradigm of dementia survival with dignity, walking with you on that journey from diagnosis to death.

We people with dementia are looking towards new horizons of hope, as we seek liberation from internalizing the oppressor of dementia.

As persons with dementia, we can relate so well to what Nelson Mandela said in his inaugural speech: 'As we let our own light shine, we unconsciously give other people permission to do the same. As we are liberated from our own fear, our presence automatically liberates others!'[11]

To live with 'the fear of ceasing to be' takes enormous courage. The precious string of pearls, of memories, that is our life, is breaking; the pearls are being lost. But by finding new pearls, those created in the struggle with dementia, we can put together a new necklace of life, of hope in our future.

We need to express our voice together, from our different perspectives of this interdependent struggle to live with the unpredictability and irrationality of dementia.

We seek a new paradigm of dementia survival with dignity, walking with you on that journey from diagnosis to death.

---

11 Commonly attributed to Mandela in error at the time this presentation was given, this quote actually comes from Marianne Williamson (1992) *A Return to Love*. London: HarperCollins, p.190.

3

An insider's view of dementia

What it is like to have dementia and what you can do to help us

Christine Bryden

October 2003[1]

My talk is about dementia from an insider's view. I have fronto-temporal dementia and will draw on my own experience, as well as that of my friends with this and other forms of dementia, to tell you what our journey with this illness is like.

As a person with dementia, I am unusual as a speaker. So often people diagnosed with a dementia, such as Alzheimer's, do not want to tell everyone what is wrong with them.

There is such a terrible stigma attached to this disease that no one wants to talk about it or admit to a diagnosis, or even seek one. So we struggle to remain 'normal' and pretend we are OK. But we are not OK. It feels very different now to how we once felt. We know what it felt like to be normal, and that is not what it feels like now. And, as the disease progresses, it becomes more and more difficult to describe how we feel, to get our thoughts in order and actually get the words out so you can understand us.

In this talk I try to describe to you what our new world is like, and how you, in the world we have now left, can help us to cope with our increasing difficulties in our daily lives. So how did it all start for me?

---

1   Plenary presentation to the ADI 19th Biennial Conference, Santo Domingo, October 2003, delivered also in amended form at events in India, Israel, South Africa, Brazil, Taiwan and Japan that year. Subsequently presented on many occasions by request in substantially revised and updated form in Australia, Japan, and mid-Indian Ocean (on a cruise ship). This is the latest version, with an MRI (magnetic resonance imaging) scan from 2011.

Becoming a labelled person

Problems since 1988.

Medical tests in 1995.

Living in fear and shame.

Isolated by stigma.

I had headaches and confusion, getting lost and stressed, probably beginning in about 1988. But all of this I thought was because of my stressful job and personal circumstances. Finally, I had brain scans in 1995 to see why I had headaches, and these showed lots of brain damage, sufficient to diagnose dementia. I was only 46 years old – far too young, I thought.

The day before my diagnosis, I was a busy and successful divorced mother of three girls, with a high-level job with the Australian Government. The day after, I was a label: Person with Dementia. No one knew what to say, what to expect of me, how to talk to me and whether to even visit me. I had become a labelled person, defined by my disease overnight. It was as if I had a target painted on my forehead, shouting out for all the world to see that I was blindfolded, no longer able to function in society.

My first two years were a struggle of living a life transformed by this label of dementia. I felt shame and retreated from society. This isolation is often the result of the stigma of having dementia. There was little support for someone with dementia; it was all directed towards carers. I had a terrible fear about my future: how would it feel to die with this disease?

My book...

Who am I?

- ‣ Denier
- ‣ Victim
- ‣ Realist

Who will I be when I die?

- ‣ Emotional being
- ‣ Spiritual self

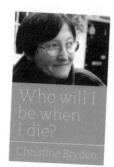

I was encouraged to write about these feelings, and wrote my first book *Who will I be when I die?*[2] in the first two years after diagnosis. My biggest fear was the later stages when I will not know who I am, who my family and friends are – and maybe even not know God.

Fear can transform us into deniers, when we pretend we are well and nothing is wrong. This pretence protects us from our fears. And our family and friends deny there is a problem, as a defence against their own feelings of grief and anger. Or fear can make us victims, so that we give up trying to function. And our family and friends adopt the new identity of carers, smothering us with their concerns and taking over our daily lives. But we can find a better way of reacting with realism to the diagnosis, by reflecting on the totality of who we are. We are far more than a cognitive self:

- We are emotional beings with relationships in this world with others.
- We are spiritual selves in relationship with the divine.

Although I appear quite normal perhaps, there is startling evidence that all is not right with me.

---

2   Christine Bryden (2012) *Who will I be when I die?* London: Jessica Kingsley Publishers (first published 1998).

My 2011 MRI scan (on left)

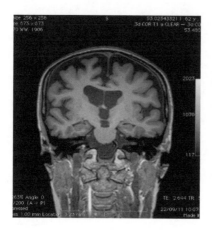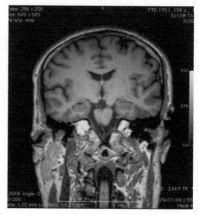

My 2011 MRI scan on the left – compared with an age-matched normal scan on the right – gave my neurologist in Sydney quite a shock! He was not prepared for such brain damage after talking to me beforehand. Apparently, these scans are consistent with moderate dementia and he would not have expected me to function very well at all, let alone speak.

The scan is a potent symbol of a life transformed by a pathology of dementia. Neurological tests simply confirmed what could be seen so clearly on this scan. Follow-up tests of all sorts over the years have shown a steady – thankfully slow – but inexorable decline in my functioning. But my brain pathology does not define me, although it is part of the curse of medical prognosis.

NOTHING ABOUT US, WITHOUT US!

My scan is my curse – a symbol of a life transformed

It led to the 'dementia script': 'You have about five years till you're demented, then about three years till death.'

Biology is not the only determinant of function, nor of my humanity.

Why do we believe the stereotype?

I was told back in 1995 the standard dementia script: 'You have about five years till you are really demented, then about three years after that in care before you die.' This is like a hospice in slow motion. But I'm still here, still talking. Biology is not the sole determinant of my function, nor of my humanity. In what way has this damaged brain made me biologically inferior? In what way am I just a brain and not a whole person?

Why are people with dementia still shunned by society, denied respect and dignity, left to retreat in shame? Why do people who come into my home to help me say, 'You don't look like you have dementia'? How am I meant to look? I still need help, and even more so as I struggle daily to cope and try to mask the difficulties I am having. Why does everyone believe in the stereotype of the dementia script, despite each of us being unique human beings in very different environments, of differing backgrounds and abilities?

Treatment delayed is treatment denied

Drugs at diagnosis slow functional decline.

I still seem normal due to my Exelon patch, as well as my previous ability.

It's like I used to juggle more balls than most, and still can keep a few in the air!

Why are many of us not offered treatment? Often we are just told the diagnosis and given no hope. At the moment of diagnosis, please give us anti-dementia medication such as Aricept, Reminyl or Exelon. These can slow down our decline. They help what remains to work better, but they do not stop the damage. It is vital to take medication as early as possible. Remember: treatment delayed is treatment denied.

My functioning seems OK because of my Exelon patch, without which I could not travel or talk. But also my previous level of education and ability help a great deal. My neurologist said it is as if I used to juggle six balls, whereas ordinary people juggled three at most. I have dropped maybe four balls now because of the brain damage, but I still juggle almost as many balls as the ordinary person I meet each day. Importantly, though, this means I can still speak and tell you what it feels like to have dementia. I have a huge battle each day with the decline from this disease, despite an apparent level of remaining function. I can share with you the journey from diagnosis into further decline.

So what does it feel like?

My identity crisis

‣ Who am I?

My environment is vital

‣ Where am I?

My daily struggle

‣ How can I cope?

Our first thoughts after diagnosis often turn to who we are and who we will become. We face an identity crisis. We have fear of the future, fear of decline, fear of death in a state of unknowing.

We can no longer be defined by our work, our contribution to the community, but have a new identity thrust upon us as a diseased person – no longer valued by society, no longer needed for making any contribution. We are very susceptible to our environment:

- If you do everything for us, we will rapidly forget functions.
- If you don't listen to us, we may give up the struggle to speak.
- If you put us in confusing or noisy surroundings, we may find it too hard to focus.

We face a daily struggle to cope. Each day is filled with a myriad of activities which become more and more difficult as time goes by. Our life becomes fragmented, as each task seems bigger and more overwhelming, so that we lose the interconnectedness of our thread of life.

We face an identity crisis

Fear of future decline.

Stigma and isolation.

Enable us to live a new life in the slow lane of dementia:

- ‣ acknowledge our disability and help us function
- ‣ focus on what we can still do, not what we can no longer do.

In our crisis of identity, we need you to acknowledge who we are, to listen to our emotion and pain, and to treat us as people of value and dignity, worthy of respect.

- The fear of future decline is a terrible thing to live with. It's a curse that leads to its own fulfilment. Give us hope.

- Understand and help us through our depression, anger, grief and loss. Try to help us overcome shame and isolation.

- Include us in all your activities, visit us and just be with us if you do not know what to say. We don't need words so much as your presence, your sharing with us of feelings.

- Do what you can to prevent the stigma of dementia. Stigma leads to shame and isolation, and a lack of treatment and support. As people with dementia, we need to be free of stigma in order to feel respected and empowered.

- Please don't say, 'That always happens to me!' or 'I feel like that, too.' This demeans us in our daily struggle to cope.

But you can enable us to live a new life in the slow lane of dementia, by acknowledging our disease and resultant disability, and doing all you can to help us function, focusing on what we can still do, not what we can no longer do.

We are much more than a diseased brain

Psychic resources.

Personality.

Environment:

- avoid noise

- have routine

- how you talk to us, not what you say

- listen carefully so we feel valued.

We are so much more than our diseased brain! We each have a unique personality that will shine through – again, with your help and encouragement.

We can draw on our inner psychic resources to cope with this new challenge to our daily life. We have our life story, which tells how we coped in the past. And this affects how we can cope today. Now we need your help even more to do so.

Most importantly, our environment will have a big impact on how we function with dementia. You can do a great deal to help by managing our environment. Avoid background noise, which will make me tired and confused. Please don't play music or have the TV on when you are talking to me.

Encourage routine so that we feel safe in a familiar environment, with activities that we can recall, so reducing the stress of making sense of our surroundings.

As we become more emotional and less cognitive, it's the way you talk to us, not what you say, that we will remember. We know the feeling but don't know the plot. Your smile, your laugh and your touch are what we will connect with.

We need you to listen carefully as we can't repeat our words. We struggle to speak and it often comes out in a very scrambled way, without proper grammar and syntax. Please try to hear the feelings we are trying to convey. Being listened to will make us feel valued and in a relationship with you. This is what we need as we cope with shattered thoughts and fragmented selves.

So what does it feel like?

Juggling and struggling

Kaleidoscope of problems, like impossible juggling of multitude of struggles:

▸ doing daily tasks

▸ speaking thoughts

▸ writing words

▸ reading stories

▸ calculating numbers.

Life has become a fragmented kaleidoscope of problems as we juggle an enormous pile of difficult tasks. We feel as if we are hanging on to a cliff, above a lurking black hole.

Daily tasks are complex. Nothing is automatic any more. Everything is as if we are first learning. Cooking burns, ironing is forgotten, washing is no longer sorted, and driving becomes scary.

As we speak, gaps in the flow of words appear. In our head a string of pictures has formed, but the words for those pictures no longer make their way into our consciousness, let alone to our mouth. And we might forget what we wanted to say just as we open our mouth – so we gape like a fish sometimes.

Our writing looks odd. And if we want to jot down something that we have just thought of, again the idea often disappears before we can even put pen to paper. It's so frustrating!

Reading a book or following a story on TV is another struggle, as we cannot recognize the faces or names, nor remember the plot as it unfolds.

Calculating has become another hurdle. We struggle to write numbers, line them up and do simple arithmetic. We don't always remember what we are supposed to do.

If we had an arm or leg missing, you would congratulate us on our efforts. But you cannot see how much of our brain is missing and how hard it is to cope, so you don't understand our struggles.

Living in a fog

- ‣ Confusion.
- ‣ Tiredness.
- ‣ Memory loss.
- ‣ Emotion.

For me it's like living in a fog, especially without my Exelon patch. Everything is confusing, and the struggle is exhausting to the point of extreme tiredness.

I have lost the map in my head, or at least the way it connects to reality around me. So I need you to guide me around, unless I am in very familiar places in the area around my house. Maybe a few prompts such as left, right, straight ahead.

I have an erratic memory. Some days I can remember this morning, but on other days I can't. It's as if I have lost all but one remaining key to the filing cabinet of my memories. You can help me try to retrieve a memory by finding a word, or a sentence, or a description of the event.

Questions like 'Do you remember?' will make me panic. The black curtain falls down behind me as I desperately try to search for some recollection connecting to what you are asking. Descriptions of your own recollections are much more helpful, as these create a word picture into which I can walk and try to recapture my own memory.

I usually enjoy each moment of our time together, so why is it so important that I remember it? Please keep visiting me, even if I might not remember you came before, or even who you are. The emotion of your visit and the friendly feelings you give to me are far more important.

It is the emotion I connect to, not the cognitive awareness of the event. I enjoy my moments of wellbeing, even if I have forgotten them later.

Stressed, restless and manic

- Agitation and anxiety.
- Apathy or focus.
- Paranoia and delusions.
- 'An abnormal reaction to an abnormal situation is normal behavior.'

As emotional beings, we feel buffeted by our environment, with few cognitive resources to cope with stress. We often feel agitated and anxious. It's as if something terrible might happen, but we have forgotten what it is.

With the stress of many activities at once, I become very focused, trying with all the brain I have left to concentrate. Telling me to rest won't help, but helping me to complete the task will.

Panic attacks and mania come upon us like storms, expressing an inner conflict as we desperately try to cope with not knowing what has happened, what is happening and what will happen. Please help us and give us a break from the effort of coping.

Another way for us to deal with stress is apathy – to switch off, because of overload. There is simply too much happening at once to bother to try to cope. It's not a lack of interest, but a lack of energy.

Paranoia and delusions are a natural part of us trying to make sense of an increasingly confusing and stressful environment. We create our own stories to explain what is happening. We become non-diplomatic, focused on our own firmly held beliefs as to what is happening around us.

As Victor Frankl has said: 'An abnormal reaction to an abnormal situation is normal behavior.'[3] Our behaviour is normal, considering what is happening inside our heads. Try to enter our distorted reality, because if you try to make us fit in with your reality, it will cause extra stress.

---

3   Viktor E. Frankl (1985) *Man's Search for Meaning*, New York: Washington Square Press, p.38.

NOTHING ABOUT US, WITHOUT US!

Sleep, dreams and reality

Dreams become vivid.

- ▸ What is dream?
- ▸ What is reality?

Sleep eludes us.

- ▸ Like jet lag.
- ▸ Can't switch brain off.

Hallucinations and illusions.

Our reality can become caught between dreams and daily life. Dreams are very vivid, because our sleeping mind is trying to master the waking confusion resulting from our damaged brain and our high level of emotions. Our dreams are so real that it is difficult to recall what is dream and what is not.

Yet dreams can be elusive, while we toss and turn waiting for sleep. Dementia disturbs the circadian rhythm of our bodies, so it feels like permanent jet lag. We cannot find the switch to turn off our brain. Warm milk, a warm bath or relaxing music may help.

I find that visualizing calm places in my mind, or praying, as I wait for sleep is increasingly difficult. I can no longer hold on to images or words in my head. It all becomes a muddle of emotions bubbling up from what has happened through the day, so increasing my stress.

Some of us find animals – real or stuffed – help us to visualize concepts such as peace, hope, faith, comfort. Touching their reality can soothe us in this struggle for sleep, as well as in the struggle to know we are awake.

But a stuffed animal can cause alarm! We can mistake what we see so easily. It's as if lots of pixels are missing, so we try to make up a picture from a blurred image. My friend, who also has dementia, muffled a scream at the dead cat in his shopping trolley. But then he realized it was his own fur hat!

Our brains try to make sense of what we see, but it is not always real.

What are the keys for coping?

▸ Faith.

▸ Paul, my 'enabler'.

▸ Medication.

▸ Attitude.

To cope in this confusing reality is a daily struggle. My keys for coping are a strong Christian faith, Paul my enabler, my Exelon and a positive attitude.

Our faith, or our spirituality, is crucial. We are losing our cognitive self – even a reliable and coherent emotional self. What remains is our spirituality. We need you to help us connect to whatever has given us true meaning in life, whether this is faith, nature or art.

Family and friends can gives us an oasis of emotional warmth in an otherwise confusing world. You are our enablers on this journey, and we need you to meet our needs as we become less and less able to deal with this illness.

Medication such as Exelon is important to clear the fog. It gives me the ability to speak and to remain aware of and concerned about what is happening around me. Without it, I am apathetic, unable to cope with daily life. Other anti-dementia medications include Aricept, Reminyl and Memantine.

My attitude to life and to disease has had a big impact. As Pastor Charles Swindoll has said, life is 10 per cent what actually happens to us, and 90 per cent how we react to it. All of us can choose our attitude each day.

Choosing to be a survivor

Connect across the divide between your world and mine.

Let's transform personal tragedy into triumph.

Let's inject new meaning and dignity into the veins of civilization.

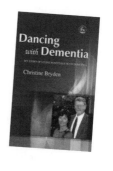

I choose a new identity as a survivor. I want to live positively each day, in a vital relationship of trust with my enabler, Paul, alongside me. Each step in this journey with dementia is like a dance in which the music is constantly changing. You can help us by adjusting your steps to the discordant music of dementia, and enabling us to cope with this confusing and ever-changing dance.

Like Viktor Frankl, we people with dementia want to be able to 'bear witness to the uniquely human potential at its best, which is to transform a personal tragedy into a triumph'.[4]

You can help us by listening to us, by giving us sensitive feedback, by acknowledging our feelings and respecting us as people of value and worth. Don't demean us by saying you know what it feels like. How can you unless you share this disease?

We know what it feels like to be normal, and that is not what it is like now. We have stepped into this new world of dementia. It is as if we are bicultural and have stepped across the divide between your world and ours.

With your understanding and support, we can help you to help us. We can make history together.

In Martin Luther King's words, let's together become a people who injected a new meaning into the veins of history and of civilization.[5]

Thank you.

---

4   Viktor E. Frankl (1985) *Man's Search for Meaning,* New York: Washington Square Press, p.135.
5   Speech to Montgomery Improvement Association 5 December 1955, available at http://kingencyclopedia. stanford.edu/encyclopedia/documentsentry/the_addres_to_the_first_montgomery_improvement_association_mia_mass_meeting, accessed on 1 July 2015.

Dementia diagnosis from an 'insider's' perspective

There is no time to lose!

Christine Bryden

August 2004[1]

I want to thank Alzheimer's Australia (Queensland) for giving me this opportunity to speak to you today, as an advocate of people with dementia.

There are more of us being diagnosed each day with dementia, and we are receiving early diagnosis and treatment, so we are less likely to fit your stereotype of a person in the later stages of these diseases. We are able to express our needs, and we want you to listen to us.

There is no time to lose to listen to our voice, to hear the 'insider's' perspective of what it is like to live with dementia, and what support we need. We have very little time to influence your policies and programs, as we struggle with this progressive terminal illness.

However, sometimes we cannot join Alzheimer associations, as they arose from the carers' movement some years ago. But why should people with dementia, as consumers of these associations' services and support, be excluded from full and equal participation? Surely it is unethical to collect and distribute funds for services on our behalf, without regard for our dignity?

---

1   Presented at the Nurses in Management of Aged Care (NIMAC) Annual Conference, Gold Coast, August 2004. The 'Christine Bryden Award' was inaugurated at this conference, offering free registration for five Aged Care Nurses in Training. Nine years later, Christine was honoured to present the annual awards at the NIMAC Conference in 2013. The talk was also given at the launch of Alzheimer's Australia Queensland (Incorporated) (AAQ), in 2004, and to several other organizations.

A recent report spoke of the dementia epidemic in Australia: there were more than 162,000 people with dementia last year, and by 2040 there will be half a million.[2] Just think of the impact on individuals, the health care system and the economy!

Until there is a cure, we are on a one-way road from diagnosis to death, and we need your support.

---

2 Beginning in 2003, Alzheimer's Australia commissioned a number of reports from Deloitte Access Economics to research and produce estimates of the current and future impact of dementia in Australia.

Advocacy

Alzheimer's Australia is a world leader.

Alzheimer's Disease International taking up the challenge.

Alzheimer's Australia (Queensland) part of global movement.

I have recently been elected to the Board of Alzheimer's Disease International for a term of three years. I am the first person with dementia on the Board. But I cannot become a member of my local association in my own right, unless I say I am part of the family of the carer. Why is this so? Maybe this is because there are two views of people with dementia:

1. either we fit the stereotype so do not have insight or capacity to make a contribution, or

2. we communicate effectively, so cannot possibly have dementia.

This is a challenge to Alzheimer's Australia (Queensland) and its member associations, which are now part of the national and global dementia movement.

Our national Alzheimer's Australia is one of the world leaders in its approach to the inclusion of people with dementia and their families in all aspects of developing national policies and programs.

Alzheimer's Disease International has followed this lead and is addressing this issue of human rights for people with dementia. We are to be heard, and we are to be included.

Where does our journey start?

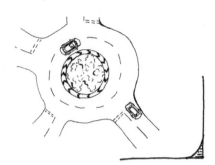

- ‣ Confusion…
- ‣ Tiredness…
- ‣ Stress…

Life's like a confusing roundabout!

My talk is a personal one, about being diagnosed with dementia in 1995.

So what is it like for us, and where does our journey start? The first signs of dementia are very gradual changes in ourselves, so that we hardly notice them. Our family and friends might think we are 'not ourselves', and we might think we are just stressed. But it is the beginning of a long slow journey of change.

I felt foggy in my head and became more readily confused. It was like this picture of cars everywhere at the roundabout. I could not work out what to do sometimes. I was very tired, and just wanted to come home from work and sleep. But I couldn't give up and go to bed. I was a recently divorced mother with three girls to look after at home, as well as 30 staff and a budget of several million Australian dollars to worry about at work.

I was so stressed out by ordinary things and was getting terrible migraines every week. I would forget things in mid-sentence, get confused about finding my way to work and found it increasingly difficult to make decisions. It really was a confusing roundabout of work and home life. Everything was an effort, and something felt very wrong! Finally, we pluck up the courage, or our family persuades us, to go to the doctor. And the journey towards diagnosis begins.

The trials of testing

- ‣ Neuropsychological tests.
- ‣ Brain scans.
- ‣ Other tests.
- ‣ Fear and dread.
- ‣ Embarrassment.
- ‣ Clinging to the hope that it can be cured!

Sometimes we have just a Mini Mental State Examination, and get the date, spelling or counting wrong and we are very embarrassed. Or we have difficult psychometric tests from a clinical psychologist. We know something is wrong, and just hope that no one notices just how much slower and confused we are now.

I came home from the testing absolutely exhausted, and puzzled as to why some things had seemed so hard and yet others quite easy. I had great difficulty remembering numbers, making pictures into a story, working out what was so special about arrangements of blocks set out before me, and making my way through a maze. My mind was often blank when trying to recall the various shopping lists and stories.

The various brain scans were very scary. Needles were sometimes stuck in my arms. Other times I was strapped to a steel table and wheeled into a thing that looked like a torpedo tube, and some of the machines sounded like roadworks. I felt trapped inside, all alone, unable to speak or move for what seemed like hours, and then was extremely confused as I tried to find my way back to my clothes and to the waiting room.

While we wait for the results, we feel fear, dread and embarrassment. What if it is dementia? How terrible to be like those people in nursing homes who wander about and don't know who they are! We hope desperately it is something that can be cured.

> While we wait for the results, we feel fear, dread and embarrassment.

Black and white reality of a scan

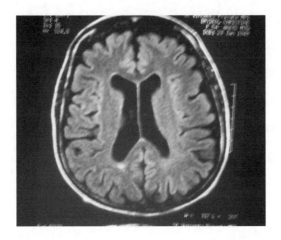

But the scans present an awful reality to us in black and white.

This Magnetic Resonance Imaging (MRI) scan of my brain was taken in November 2003, eight years after diagnosis. It shows more damage than the scans in May 2001 and May 1995.

At first I tried desperately to believe that the damage had always been there. Maybe I had been born with that amount of brain missing and coped very well despite it.

But now, as these regular
scans chart slow but
inexorable tissue loss,
I must face the reality of
progressive brain damage.

The 'dementia script'!

'You have dementia.'

'There is no cure.'

'You have about five years till you are "demented" and then you can expect to live another three years.'

The time of tests is an agony of waiting, wondering and desperately hoping that whatever is wrong can be treated and life can go back to normal.

But life changes dramatically. We face the shock of diagnosis.

It feels like a curse when the doctor says, 'You have dementia. There is no cure.' It's like the pointing-bone of a traditional curse, and what is said often leads to a terrible depression.

Many of us have heard at diagnosis what we now refer to as the standard dementia script: 'You have about five years till you become demented; then you'll probably die about three years later.'

No wonder we often suffer depression and despair!

Many of us wish we had cancer. At least then usually there is talk of treatment, of chemotherapy, of possible remission. There is none of that with a diagnosis of dementia. People with dementia have compared what we heard at diagnosis. It was the same script, yet we are all such different people, with different diseases, different personalities and ways of coping.

No wonder we often suffer depression and despair!

How come the doctors all around the world tell us the same prognosis?

Shock of diagnosis and horror of prognosis

A turning point…

- trauma, disbelief or relief.

Awful awareness of future –

- our world has collapsed,

- everything has changed.

We face a defeat of spirit and of hope!

The dementia script – the shock of diagnosis and horror of prognosis – is a turning point in our lives. That moment is etched in our memories. What the weather was like, what people were wearing and what people said emerge from the fog of our distorted memories as one crystal-clear picture.

For some of us, it is a relief. At last there is an explanation for our confusion, slowness, memory loss and daily difficulties. But we still must face up to what the future now holds.

For others, diagnosis leads to disbelief. There is nothing wrong with us, surely! No one can think we are anything like those people in nursing homes who don't know who they are or who their families are?

And for others, like me, it is a time of trauma. I faced an awful awareness of my future, of what lay ahead for me and for my girls. I would have to stop work and would still need to support the family. My world had collapsed. Everything had changed. I faced a defeat of spirit and of hope.

Our identity crisis

Loss of identity.

- ‣ Who am I?
- ‣ Will anyone respect me?
- ‣ Who will I be when I die?

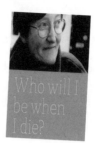

Our main fear is the 'loss of self' associated with dementia. We face an identity crisis. We all believe the toxic lie of dementia: that the mind is absent and the body is an empty shell. Our sense of self is shattered with this new label of dementia.

Who am I if I can no longer be a valued member of society? What if I don't know my family, if I don't know who I am and who I was, if I don't even know God? These concerns led me to write a book *Who will I be when I die?*,[3] reprinted several times since then and now released in Japanese and Chinese, and in the USA.

We can find a new identity as an emotional being. We can hug, we can have cuddly toys once more, we can cry and express pain more freely. In our relationships we connect at a deeper level.

We have inner psychic resources that arise from our personality and life story. These resources – our attitude – affect how we cope with brain damage. If we give up, we appear to have a greater degree of dementia.

And, importantly, each of us has a spiritual self. Even without words for the pictures in our mind, we can find meaning in life in our own spirituality. My Christian faith, my spiritual relationship with God through Jesus, can flourish as an important source of my identity.

But what about our families?

---

3   Christine Bryden (2012) *Who will I be when I die?* London: Jessica Kingsley Publishers (first published 1998).

We both become victims…

I thought my world would end.

A mix of emotions…fear, dread.

Didn't know much about dementia.

Our families feel distress and shock at the diagnosis. But there are various ways in which they react to the trauma.

One way is to focus on how their own future is in tatters. Their world has collapsed around them, so that both the person with dementia and the family become victims.

My youngest daughter was only nine at the time of my diagnosis. She was not able to understand what dementia meant and did not have the emotional resources to deal with the trauma. Now 18, she says:

> I thought my world would end. I didn't know what emotions to feel –
> fear, dread – and what I was going to see as I didn't know much about
> dementia. At first I went 'off the rails', as I didn't't know how to deal with
> the diagnosis.

Then, with information and love, a coping strategy can evolve. For my youngest daughter this has taken some years, as she deals with these emotions during her teenage years. Now she is able to say:

> I realized Mum would still be the same and I would still love her, although
> it would hurt me to see her decline. So I got myself back together, and
> wanted to make sure I had a special relationship with Mum, as that was
> what was important for us.

Withdrawing into denial…

I was scared…angry…to think Mum wouldn't know me.

The only way I could cope was to withdraw to my horse.

My middle daughter was 14, and is now 23. Like her younger sister, the diagnosis was a shock and brought with it fear of the future, anger about what had happened and a terrible sadness about loss.

She said:

> I was scared that I would not have a mum that knew me, and a few years later she would die. I was angry that even though she was such a firm Christian this could happen to us. Hadn't enough happened already? It was like the last straw.

Her escape from this trauma was her horse, which was a means of withdrawing from the reality of diagnosis, and to deny anything was wrong. She had become a denier and it almost seemed to me as if she did not care what was happening.

As she says now:

> The only way I could cope was to hide my emotions and withdraw into myself. Now I am older and have seen Mum still here, but changing slowly, so I have come to terms with it and want to make the most of time with Mum.

Carers, martyrs and sufferers?

I was very concerned for Mum and took care of a lot of things at home…although I 'lost it' a couple of times and cried my eyes out.

I needed to be there for her.

A more common way a family deals with the trauma of diagnosis is to suppress their own feelings of shock and loss, and to adopt the 'carer' role. My eldest daughter was 20. She became the carer, the responsible one, looking after her sisters, taking the load off me.

Now 29, she says:

> At first I felt shock and disbelief, but then was very concerned for Mum and how she would deal with this. I needed to be there for Mum, so I took a year off university and looked after my sisters, helped Mum with an Enduring Power of Attorney, and took care of a lot of things at home.

Her emotions were held in check as she coped as a carer. But every now and then her emotions spilled out in times of crying, when she wept over my loss as well as her own. As she says:

> I had to keep going. But I 'lost it' a couple of times and cried my eyes out, because it was so tragic for Mum. She had just got divorced and had a very stressful life.

Often I see families who smother us with care as they adopt this 'carer' role, becoming a martyr and sacrificing their own needs for ours. This martyr complex limits us both, as the only identity the family has is as a carer, and our only role is as a sufferer. We fade as we withdraw from trying, and you burn out from trying too hard.

Care-partner

Not smothered by your care, nor isolated by your denial,
nor cast aside as a victim of your grief.

But a care-partner walking alongside to meet our increasing needs.

There is a balance to become a care-partner. The person with dementia is not smothered by your care, nor isolated by your denial, nor cast aside as a victim of your grief. You walk alongside us as we struggle to cope with diminishing functions and increasing emotions.

When I met Paul in 1998 through an introductions agency, and told him about my diagnosis three years before, he was very pragmatic and said, 'I can cope with that.' We got married a year later, and he is still able to cope today, despite me having lost a great deal of function.

He loves me for who I really am, not for my cognitive function alone, but also for my emotions and spirituality with which I can connect with others.

Paul's view is that it is best to help and encourage me to do as much as I can while I can. Sometimes it feels as if I have to struggle too hard with not enough care; other times there is too much help. It is a fine balance, but a care-partner, rather than a carer, helps me to maintain function for longer.

We need you to read our mind, watch our coping ability and adjust your caring in accord with our need, which will increase gradually along this journey from diagnosis to death.

But a major concern for us and our family, our care-partners, is the stigma that surrounds us.

Stigma of dementia – social isolation

Myths and fears about dementia lead to stigma.

This gives us a 'degenerating sense of "nobodiness"'
(Martin Luther King).

We are isolated by the stigma or dementia.

The myths and fears about dementia – the stereotype of someone in the later stages of the diseases that cause dementia – lead to a social stigma which affects all of our social interactions.

You say we do not remember, so we cannot understand. We do not know, so it is OK to distance yourself from us. And this leads to our isolation, as you treat us with fear and dread. The stigma isolates us in our encounters with family and friends. We cannot work, we cannot drive, we cannot contribute to society.

I am watched carefully for signs of odd words or behaviour, my opinion is no longer sought, and I am thought to lack insight, so it does not matter that I am excluded. We know what it feels like to have the 'degenerating sense of "nobodiness"'[4] that oppressed Martin Luther King's fellow black Americans.

The diagnosis of dementia has changed our world forever.

---

4   Martin Luther King, Jr (2010) Why We Can't Wait. Boston, MA: Beacon Press (first published 1964), p.88.

But there is hope!

- ▸ Inform us.
- ▸ Give us treatment.
- ▸ Offer legal help.
- ▸ Offer emotional support.
- ▸ Encourage us to be positive.
- ▸ We can reach for the stars together!

But there is hope after a diagnosis of dementia. It is possible to live positively.

Information is important and empowering. Tell us about the diagnosis, about how little is known and how individual each one of us is.

Offer **treatment** immediately, because function that we lose is not easily regained. I have been taking Aricept since mid-2000 and now have the Exelon patch. Without this, it is like thinking in fog and walking in treacle. Life is a confusing daze, like the roundabout on my second slide.

Offer **legal help**, because we need to know that we have a terminal illness, so we can get our affairs in order. I arranged an Enduring Power of Attorney, giving me peace of mind.

We need **emotional support**, especially immediately after diagnosis. Listen to our anger and grief, and help us deal with emotional issues from the past and grief at what we will lose in the future. Individual counselling and support groups will help.

Most importantly, **encourage us to be positive**, to hope for a new life in the slow lane, as we reach for the stars together.

Making music with what's left

We celebrate a new life in the slow lane, as we try to find the pearls within us.

Our attitude transforms the pattern of our life, so we are no longer victims but survivors.

We can find out how much music we can still make with what we have left, as we celebrate this new life in the slow lane. We can find new ways to enjoy each moment of our day. For me it is the joy of sunshine, of seeing flowers and sunsets, and of stroking cats and hugging my husband.

We can develop new talents – the pearls hidden within us – by focusing on relationships and greater emotional connection, rather than on cognition. We can also rediscover our spirituality, developing a greater awareness of what gives us meaning in life. My Christianity certainly flourished, as I turned to my faith in anger, fear, confusion – and eventually acceptance.

Our attitude transforms the pattern of our life, and we can choose to live positively with dementia, through drawing on our inner psychic resources and our spirituality to view each day, each hour, as a gift.

Through this we are no
longer victims, but survivors.

NOTHING ABOUT US, WITHOUT US!

Sharing our insights on this journey from diagnosis to death

Listen to our broken voices and our fragmented memories.

Let's work together as equal partners on the journey.

There is no time to lose.

As survivors of the journey with dementia, we can share with you the insider's knowledge that we have. But you need to ask us, and you need to include us.

We have confronted a living death, and we are still trying to find ways to liberate ourselves from this fear of ceasing to be. We know what it was once like to be normal, like you. We know both your world and ours. There is a great deal we could share with you, if you could only include us as equal partners with you on this journey with dementia.

Find a way to listen to our broken voices, our disjointed thoughts and our fragmented memories of how things are and used to be. Let's work together to share our insights as equal partners – people with dementia, their families, and those who support them – on this journey from diagnosis to death. There is no time to lose.

Thank you.

5

Dancing with dementia

Christine Bryden

October 2004[1]

This talk covers the main aspects of my new book *Dancing with Dementia*.[2] It takes you on through the many twists and turns of the journey of my life since 1998, when my first book *Who will I be when I die?*[3] was published.

The book describes how I began studies, was re-diagnosed and met Paul, all in the same year. It also tells the story of how a group of people with dementia got together on the internet and managed to change things by acting locally and thinking globally. The book describes what it feels like to have dementia and what you can do to help, and answers many frequently asked questions.

I reflect on my journey of understanding, of seeing more clearly who I am now, who I am becoming and who will I be when I die. Looking back, it has been an amazing journey of self-discovery, change and growth.

I have learned how to dance with dementia, how to adapt to change, how to express my needs and how to stay in tune with the music as it slows.

I plan to continue this dance with dementia to my full potential, with Paul alongside me as my dance partner, my care-partner on this journey.

---

1 Delivered at Yokohama and Tokyo, while launching *Dancing with Dementia*, in October 2004.
2 Christine Bryden (2005) *Dancing with Dementia: My Story of Living Positively with Dementia*. London: Jessica Kingsley Publishers.
3 Christine Bryden (2012) *Who will I be when I die?* London: Jessica Kingsley Publishers (first published 1998).

A roller-coaster ride

I began studies in counselling, struggling but doing well.

But I battled depression, despite believing that I was getting better.

Was I overcoming depression? Or was the disease slowing down, or even stopping?

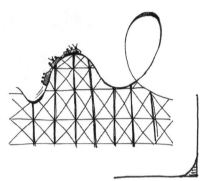

My journey so far has been like a roller-coaster ride, with me hanging on to the little cart as it hurtles up and down the rails. All sorts of things have happened that I never dreamed were possible when I wrote my first book.

In early 1998, while the first book was still at the publishers, I began studies for a post-graduate diploma in counselling. It was like the long slow haul up one side of the roller-coaster, as I struggled to cope with learning new things, doing essays and searching the internet. The studies went very well, and soon it felt as if I was rushing down the other side of the roller-coaster, towards gaining a better understanding of how people with dementia could be supported in groups and individually. By 2002 I had published a literature review based on my studies.

During this time, though, I battled depression, because of the medical prognosis that had been given to me in 1995 – that I would be demented in about five years and then be in a nursing home for a few years before dying of dementia. Yet I had faith in being able to stay well for longer than expected, in being able to help others who had been diagnosed with dementia and in being able to live life to the full.

I believed that I was getting better, not as confused, not as slow. Was this because of overcoming depression? Or was it really because the disease process was slowing down or even stopping?

I'm really getting better!

Neurological reassessment scans and psychometric tests.

Either I was getting better, remaining stable, declining, or maybe it was all just a figment of my imagination.

But he said my disease looked like a 'glacially slow' dementia of the fronto-temporal type.

So I went to the neurologist for a check-up. I told him that I felt I was really getting better, but he said, 'Make the most of this temporary honeymoon.'

However, he did order more tests, including computerized tomography, radio nuclide brain perfusion and positron emission tomography scans, as well as extensive psychometric tests.

This neurological reassessment was going to be a 'circuit breaker' for me. Either I was getting better, remaining stable or declining. Or maybe it was all just a figment of my imagination. The neurologist would be able to see how my disease was progressing, and whether I really had a future other than decline into dementia.

It was a memorable moment when the neurologist rang me at home and said that all the tests and scans had showed that my deterioration was 'glacially slow'. He said that now my brain damage looked more like a fronto-temporal type of dementia, rather than dementia of the Alzheimer's type. Despite the equally gloomy prognosis for such a dementia, he said mine was unusually slow, and that I would live to see any grandchildren.

I was delighted and excited at this news. It meant so much to me, as by then – unbelievably – I was thinking of getting married, which in itself was an amazing twist to my roller-coaster ride of life!

A new lease of life!

I met Paul in mid-1998 and we were married a year later.

The miracle continues:

Not only am I better than I could have hoped for, but I have a loving husband who shares my strong faith and supports me as I decline with dementia.

Yes, I had gone to an introductions agency and met Paul. I speak in my new book about how we danced around the kitchen after this phone call from the neurologist, which gave us both so much hope for the future!

We had met on a chilly winter's day, in July 1998, and walked for hours around the beautiful lake in Canberra. Soon he was at my door with flowers every day, with a big smile on his face. What joy he brought into my life! We married in our church a year later, sharing our joy, faith and hope with friends and family. People who were at the wedding were overjoyed. Just four years before, when I was diagnosed, they thought they were losing me to Alzheimer's disease. Now they could see that I was still very much alive, and getting married to a lovely man.

Each day since then this miracle has continued. Not only am I better than I could have hoped for, but I have a loving husband who shares my strong faith and supports me as I decline with dementia. Even just a few years ago, and certainly while I was writing my first book, this seemed impossible.

With Paul by my side, I then began the long journey of battling the stereotype of dementia and of trying to get more support and recognition for people with dementia from the local, national and international Alzheimer's movement.

Challenging the stereotype

Battling the stereotype of dementia, of someone in the later stages.

If I could speak, I did not have dementia.

My diagnosis is still questioned.

What is it about dementia that makes people demand proof?

Why can't we cheer the dementia survivors?

The stereotype of dementia is of the later stages, of the person lacking insight and being unable to speak. The long journey beforehand – between diagnosis and the end stage, of living with dementia each day – is ignored.

With the publication of my first book *Who will I be when I die?* in 1998, I had 'come out', brave enough to admit to a disease that is feared and talking about this long journey with dementia. But I had to battle the stereotype, which had led to the exclusion of people with dementia from the activities of the Alzheimer's movement. At first I was not regarded as a credible representative. If I could speak, I did not have dementia.

My diagnosis is still repeatedly questioned. But if I had gone public with, say, a diagnosis of breast cancer, would people want to see the scars? What is it about dementia that makes people demand proof? We applaud the bravery and courage of people battling cancer. Why can't we cheer the dementia survivors? Maybe many of us would survive better and longer if we did not also have to battle against the stereotype of dementia.

Meeting my 'cyber' friends

In DASNI, people with dementia around the world shared how they felt.

I was not alone.

Together we were:

- challenging the stereotype of dementia, and
- seeking to change negative attitudes.

I felt very much alone in this battle against the stereotype of dementia, until I joined an internet-based group that later became Dementia Advocacy and Support Network International, or DASNI.

Across the globe, people with dementia shared how they felt. We were still able to communicate, willing to speak out and wanting to challenge the accepted view of the later stages of the disease. Most of us were taking anti-dementia medication, and we were not willing to accept being categorized into a medical model of decline according to set stages.

But maybe it was all too easy to hide behind our computer screens and send emails to each other about how we felt. How were we going to change the negative attitudes we faced?

The first step in the battle against the stereotype was when a DASNI friend, Morris Friedell, from the US came to Australia. Together we gave a talk at the national conference.[4] Now it was clear that I was not the only one able to speak.

The next step was in June 2001, when DASNI members gathered in Montana, in the US, and developed a proposal to Alzheimer's Disease International (ADI). We wanted people with dementia to be included locally, nationally and internationally.

> We were challenging
> the stereotype; we were
> seeking change.

---

4   See Chapter 1.

DASNI's chance to shine!

We were becoming visible.

The stereotype was being challenged.

By acting locally and thinking globally, DASNI was making an impact.

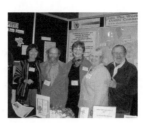

Later that year in New Zealand, at the annual ADI conference, people with dementia from Australia, New Zealand, America and Canada gathered together. As I say in the book, it was our chance to shine!

I gave a plenary address, 'Diagnosis, drugs and determination', talking about DASNI and mentioning our booth, which displayed what we were and what we stood for.

Conference attendees were baffled, intrigued and amazed. Many people involved in the global Alzheimer's movement had never met and spoken with a person with dementia. They visited our booth, took photos and began to think about their attitudes to people with dementia.

We were becoming visible, and, by doing so, the stereotype of dementia was being challenged. But it was only the beginning of the relay race towards change, and we handed on the relay baton to ADI. By 2003, we were amazed and delighted to see how the race to changing the stereotype was gaining momentum. By acting locally and thinking globally, DASNI had made an impact.

Little did I know, though, that I was to be expected to keeping running in the race, to keep hold of the baton.

Running the race

Two months of travelling.

Elected to the Board of ADI.

Settling into a new house.

Taking on the relay baton for the last leg of the relay race.

But my body was exhausted and my mind stretched beyond its meagre capacity.

In mid-2003, I had been travelling for two months, giving talks about what it feels like to have dementia. We finally arrived at the ADI conference in Santo Domingo.

It was great to meet some DASNI friends again, and I gave another plenary address. I was humbled and honoured at this conference to be elected for three years to the Board of ADI. I was the first person with dementia to be given this responsibility and accountability, and it felt as if I was taking on the baton for the last leg of the relay race.

I was overwhelmed to be trusted with this task. But what added to my feeling of exhaustion was that we arrived home to the stress of settling into the new house. My body was exhausted and my mind stretched beyond its meagre capacity. Everything felt strange and unusual.

I'm like a swan

Gliding above the water, paddling
frantically beneath the surface.

I can still swim a bit and put on a good
show, but it seems as if I will soon sink.

Nobody knows, except me and my poor
damaged brain, how bad it is.

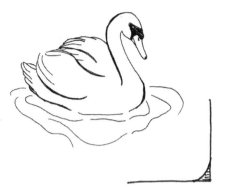

I'm like the swan, gliding above the water, paddling frantically beneath the surface. And it feels as if I am paddling faster and faster each day. It seems as if I'm going to sink soon, because the struggle is getting to the point where I feel too exhausted to keep going like this.

When I talk to the neurologist and tell him what I am doing, he sees the swan. Yet underneath, when he examines the tests and scans, he can see how fast I am paddling. I can still swim a bit and put on a good show, so that you don't notice much is wrong. Nobody knows, except me and my poor damaged brain, how bad it is.

It would be a lot easier for us just to give up, because it is a struggle every day to capture moments of clarity in the fog of our confusion. Unpredictably, we can become exhausted, confused, muddle-headed.

Struggle and anguish

Every moment of the day is a conscious effort.

The world feels like a wobbly place.

The unreliability of my memory gives such a hit-and-miss approach to life.

Every moment of the day is a conscious effort. The complexity of so many things is a source of anguish.

Stumbling, wobbling and spilling are features of daily life. The world feels like a wobbly place, and it is hard to know where each part of me is in space.

The unreliability of my memory is as if the printer ink is running low and it sometimes works and sometimes doesn't. It is such a hit-and-miss approach to life.

Black hole of a life unremembered

Muddled thoughts, with random bursts of energy and lucidity.

Intermittent reception of life as it passes by.

Living without labels, in a world in which I know that I know you, but not why I know you.

Memory comes and goes, so that there are glimpses of past events or future tasks I wish to do. It's like a 'black hole of a life unremembered'.

I have a muddle of thoughts, and try to make the most of random bursts of energy and lucidity. This intermittent reception of life as it passes by applies to what I have just asked you, too, so I ask the same question again without realizing I have asked before.

I am slowly learning how to live without remembering labels – your name, or even my name. I know faces and know I connect with them somehow, but not why I know them and what I know about them. It is a world in which I know that I know you, but not why I know you.

Anxious and out of control

We have reason to be anxious.

Was there something I promised to do or planned to do?

We are losing our way, not knowing where we are.

Communicating is difficult, so we feel frustration.

It's an exhausting way to be!

We have reason to be anxious, and we are out of control.

We cannot remember things, so we are always worried that we will lose something. We cannot remember. Was there something I promised to do? Was there something I planned to do? These thoughts spin around and get us nowhere, as we simply cannot remember. And we are losing our way, not knowing where we are.

Adding to our frustration and our anxiety is our difficulty in communicating – in reading, writing and speaking.

I struggled to write my new book, drawing on speeches, emails and media interviews, trying very hard to put it all together to make sense. It took six years to finally be able to share my thoughts collectively, slowly, reiteratively and reflectively. It is an exhausting way to be!

NOTHING ABOUT US, WITHOUT US!

How can we be helped?

Search for a cure, and:

- ▸ build on our strengths, working with reminiscence
- ▸ try to understand what this assault to our functioning is like
- ▸ manage our environment.

Find out what has given meaning to our lives: spirituality can flourish as an important source of identity.

The symptoms that we show are the result of several things working together, some of which you can address. First, there is the continuing brain damage. A cure to stop and repair this is urgently needed. I hope I last long enough to benefit.

While we wait for a cure, you can build on our strengths, working with reminiscence and, most importantly, by trying to understand what this assault to our functioning is like.

There is also plenty you can do to manage our environment. The most important way to help is finding out what has given us meaning in our lives. In the face of declining cognition and increasing emotional sensitivity, spirituality can flourish as an important source of identity.

Reach out to our spiritual self

The stigma of dementia leads to a view that we are beyond the reach of normal spiritual practices.

But you can minister to our true spiritual self.

We can find meaning in spirituality; you can connect with us and empower us.

As time passes, I will need others to understand that my odd behaviour, my lack of social graces, my lack of resources to offer in friendship do not stem from the soul that lies within me. Rather they are the product of my diseased brain.

The stigma of dementia leads to a view that we are beyond the reach of normal spiritual practices. But you can reach out to our true spiritual self that lies beyond cognition and emotion. You can help us to see beyond the transient worldly difficulties of coping each day with brain damage. Find out more about the unique individual who has dementia, about their preferences, and then find ways in which this person can be spiritually nourished. We can find meaning in our spirituality, and you can connect with us and empower us.

'Who will I be when I die?'

Dementia is described as 'loss of self'.

When do I cease being me?

We need to create a new image of who we are, and who we are becoming.

We can choose the attitude that we have.

Dementia is often described as a 'loss of self', implying that the person with dementia at some stage loses what it is to be human. But at what stage can you deny me my selfhood? Exactly when do I cease being me?

The title of my first book – *Who will I be when I die?* – reflected the fear of losing self, of a future without knowledge of identity. We face this awful fear of ceasing to be – not just a physical death, but also a gradual emotional and psychological death.

The challenge is to live in a world of hope, alternatives, growth and possibility. We need to create a new image of who we are and who we are becoming. How we do this depends very much on our personality, our life story, our health, our spirituality and our social environment.

We can choose the attitude we have.

> The challenge is to live in a world of hope, alternatives, growth and possibility.

Stripping away the masks

Dementia is a journey into the true centre of self: from cognition, through emotion, into what gives meaning in life.

If society could appreciate this, then people with dementia would be respected and treasured.

The spiritual or transcendent self remains intact through dementia.

I choose to live positively with dementia. In so doing, I am making a journey into the centre of self, away from the complex cognitive outer layer that once defined me, through the jumble and tangle of emotions created through my life experiences, into the centre of my being, into what truly gives me meaning in life.

I've begun to realize that what remains throughout this journey with dementia is what is really important, and what disappears is what is not important. I think that if society could appreciate this, then people with dementia would be respected and treasured.

Cognition is like our outer mask, our name, address, job, life story. When we remove this, we find the mask of emotions, of our relationships and feelings. These two masks become faded and scrambled with dementia. Beneath is the spiritual or transcendent self, which remains intact despite the ravages of dementia.

I'm becoming who I really am

My real self exists in the 'now', continually and eternally.

This is a new way of living, maybe even the essence of living, and is the experience of dementia.

I have answered the question of my first book.

This real self cannot exist independently in our society, which defines people by the outer layers of cognition and emotion – by our masks. It exists in the 'now', continually and eternally.

Like a bud, my true self encapsulates all the potential of what it means to be me. This is a new way of living, maybe even the essence of living, and is the experience of dementia.

I have found the answer to the question of my first book: Who will I be when I die? I'm becoming who I really am.

Dancing with dementia

I'm adapting to the ever-changing music of dementia, with my care-partner.

I'm choosing to find out how much dancing is left in me.

Much has changed since I stumbled on to this dance floor but there is still no cure, and the stereotype and stigma remain.

In my journey towards my true self, with dementia stripping away the masks of cognition and emotion, I'm choosing an attitude of dancing with dementia, to find out how much dancing is left in me.

As each decline becomes apparent, I let my care-partner, Paul, know. Together we adapt to the ever-changing music of dementia. I love the imagery of a couple dancing with dementia. It's a care-partnership, in which I am able to communicate my needs, and so be a partner in my care. We keep changing our steps in this dance to the discordant music of dementia. I desperately hope for a cure, but, in the meantime, I'll try to create and dazzle, despite my limitations.

Much has changed since I stumbled on to the dementia dance floor and Paul joined me a few years later. There is medication, there is better understanding, there is better support. But there is still no cure, and much remains to be done to challenge the stereotype and stigma of dementia.

Time is running out

My last effort to capture fleeting ideas,
to help change attitudes.

I have done all that I can.

Now it's time to rest, hoping for a cure.

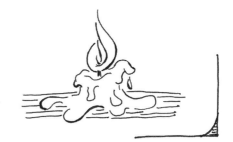

For me, time is running out. I feel like a sputtering candle, as it dies down to the last few centimetres of wax. The flame flickers just a bit more brightly before it finally disappears.

There is a stream of ideas coming through my brain, yet they don't remain there. They are fleeting glimpses of insight, there one moment, totally gone the next. My book is my last effort to capture them, to help change attitudes, to do all that I can to help others.

Now it is time to rest, and I plan to treasure each moment that remains with my family and my friends. It is time to move away from the bright lights to a corner of the dance floor where the rhythm is slower and the music quieter, but still sweet. All I can do now is sit quietly and listen, and hope for a cure.

Thank you.

6

Nothing about us, without us!

Including people with dementia

Christine Bryden

Dementia Advocacy and Support Network International (DASNI)

October 2004[1]

My talk argues that people with dementia should be given the choice for full participation in the local, national and international Alzheimer's movement. It describes how the stereotype and myth of dementia have led to the stigma that prevents people labelled with dementia from participating fully in the life of the global Alzheimer's movement. The stigma has created a barrier between people with dementia and the rest of society. This barrier is reinforced by the use of such terms as 'mindless empty shell' to gain funds and support for the global Alzheimer's movement.

As a person with dementia, and as part of the self-advocacy group DASNI, I believe that it is unethical to collect and distribute funds on behalf of disabled people without regard for our dignity. Why should people with dementia, as consumers of Alzheimer's association support and services, be excluded from full and equal participation? By becoming more visible, in all Alzheimer's association activities, with ADI as our ally, people labelled with dementia can begin to break down the barrier of stigma that denies us our humanity.

There should be nothing about us, without us, in the global Alzheimer's movement.

---

1   Presentation to a workshop on stigma at the 20th ADI Conference in Kyoto, October 2004. Christine chaired the workshop, which also had presentations from people with dementia from Canada and the UK. The session was over-subscribed, with crowds watching on large screens outside the hall. Stigma remains a major challenge.

Self-advocacy by DASNI

Started running in 2000.

Approached ADI in 2001.

Handed over the relay baton.

ADI must finish the race.

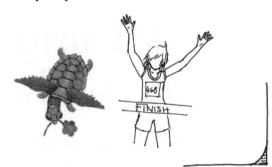

In 2000, a group of people with dementia got together over the internet to support each other in self-advocacy. We formed the Dementia Advocacy and Support Network International (DASNI).

Our logo is a winged turtle, holding a forget-me-not flower. The turtle represents our disability, our label of dementia. Its wings symbolize our desire to be set free from the stigma that prevents us from reaching our full potential. The flower is a potent reminder that we do not want to be forgotten.

DASNI approached ADI in mid-2001, seeking a greater awareness of the contribution that people with dementia could make. Like people labelled with intellectual disability, we wanted to be included, valued and appreciated as individuals.

In this relay race towards eliminating stigma, and towards self-determination, each one of us – locally, nationally, internationally – is carrying a baton of change. But, unlike people labelled with intellectual disability, we are declining daily. Not all of us in DASNI who picked up the baton and began the race in 2000 are still running. Others have now joined the race. They too will one day drop out, as they decline and become too tired to stay in the race.

Because we cannot maintain the momentum of this race towards change, DASNI has handed the relay baton of change to ADI. It is vital that ADI becomes the ally of people with dementia and runs with the baton of change to the finish line.

NOTHING ABOUT US, WITHOUT US!

What is our label?

Dementia:

- out of one's mind.

The stereotype:

- someone in the later stages.

The myth:

- we all can't speak
- we all lack insight.

Let's look at what some of the language actually means.

Dementia literally means 'out of one's mind due to brain disease or injury'. This label of dementia gives rise to a stereotype and myth which together create a wall of stigma between people with dementia and the rest of society.

A stereotype is a simplified and standardized conception of a particular group of people that is invested with special meaning. A myth is something imaginary or fictitious, and can be an unproved belief that is accepted uncritically. The stereotype of dementia is of someone in the later stages of the disease. The myth of dementia is that we are all alike, all mindless empty shells. The stereotype and myth of dementia lead to a belief that we all can't speak and that we all lack insight. We are no longer individuals with unique characteristics.

As people with dementia, we are expected to conform to society's expectations of this stereotype and myth. But most of us in DASNI do not conform to your expectations, so our activities are questioned as lacking in credibility and as not being representative of our labelled group.

We are constrained
by the stereotype and
myth of dementia.

The oppression of stigma

Stereotype and myth lead to stigma.

Society can't see the person within.

The veil of stigma masks our potential and oppresses us.

The stereotype and myth of dementia is a distorted perception that leads to stigma, which can be defined as an undesirable social property that is assigned to people when they have an attribute that deviates negatively from societal norms.

Once we are labelled with dementia, society no longer looks beyond our disability to see the person within. This stigmatizing aspect of our identity can overshadow other aspects of who we are.

The stigma of dementia leads to our exclusion from full and equal participation in the organizations that provide us with services and support. I believe that it is unethical to exclude us, as consumers, without regard for our dignity and our individuality. And without our subjective experience of living with dementia, how can policies, programs and services be better designed to meet our needs?

We people with dementia are individuals who are diverse in the nature and severity of our disability, because of our personality, our life history, the time since the onset of our disease, the type of our dementia, and our support and medication.

But what we all share is the experience of living with dementia. And what we all share, as a labelled people, is the oppression of stigma that masks our potential to participate fully in designing and modifying the services and support that we need.

Stigma is a disease of society

We are trapped within a web of stigma that:

▸ oppresses us

▸ and casts a veil across our lives.

The greater the stigma the more likely our 'adaptive behaviour'.

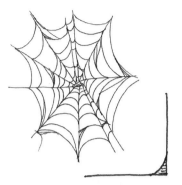

Stigma is a disease of society, adding to our disability. As people with dementia, we live within a complex web of social encounters that are tainted with stigma – like the description James Dudley uses for the stigma experienced by people with intellectual disability.[2]

Dementia is not simply a disease of the person, but is a disease of society, due to the stigma that has been created from the stereotype and myth. It seems easier for those of us who are trapped within this web to conform to the stereotype and myth, to behave in accord with the label of dementia. Society values competence, intelligence and independence, and our label – created by stereotype and myth – denies us these attributes. They are not expected of us, and not encouraged.

Labelling theory suggests that 'deviant behaviour is behaviour that people so label'.[3] So people can become what is expected of the label attached to them by society. It is also suggested that deviancy amplification can occur, where the greater the stigma, the more likely the deviant behaviour.

Perhaps stigma leads to challenging behaviour in people with dementia? Our label devalues us, we behave accordingly, and you respond. It's a reiterative cycle of reinforcing our differences.

As labelled people, we are showing what I call 'adaptive behaviour'. We are adapting to the web of stigma that entraps us, that oppresses us and casts a veil across every aspect of our lives.

2   James R. Dudley (1997) *Confronting the Stigma in Their Lives*. Springfield, IL: Charles C. Thomas.
3   Howard Becker (1963) *Outsiders: Studies in the Sociology of Deviance*. New York: Free Press of Glencoe, p.9.

How can we remove the barrier?

Stigma is a barrier behind which we experience loneliness.

We must address the stereotype and myth of dementia and focus on emotions and spirituality rather than cognition.

The stigma of dementia creates a barrier between two worlds – that of people with dementia and that of the rest of society. We are divided by the stigma associated with dementia. Behind this barrier of stigma, we experience loneliness.

We cannot meet the expectations of the world on the other side of the barrier. How can we maintain friendships with you if we are expected to remember your name, what you told us just now or what is happening in your life? You focus so much on our cognitive self, rather than trying to relate to the deeper emotional and spiritual self that each one of us shares and can connect with.

In the past, the system itself – the global Alzheimer's movement – has reinforced the barrier, by portraying us as 'mindless empty shells' in its efforts to seek funds. We need to break down this barrier, to remove the stigma, by addressing the stereotype and myth of dementia that created it. This means that we need to avoid such terms that imply all people with dementia are alike – they are all 'demented', they are all 'sufferers', they are all child-like, or all lacking in insight. We need to focus on emotions and spirituality rather than cognition, as we begin to find out ways to communicate across the barrier that divides us.

Our invisibility makes the stigma worse

When we are invisible, you believe that we are all alike.

When we become visible, we can seek a cure and treatment.

You can be our ally:

- Believe in our potential.
- You need us and we need you.

Our lack of visibility reinforces the barrier of stigma. While we remain invisible, you will continue to believe that people with dementia are all alike. We will remain trapped behind the barrier, our unique identity masked by the label of dementia.

An important way to address stigma is to include us in all of your activities and to look beyond the stigma to our living reality. By becoming visible as individuals, we can be seen as people first, before our disability. The unique purpose and meaning in each of our lives is revealed.

People with dementia want to have the choice to participate in the local, national and international Alzheimer's movement. Use us in your fundraising and awareness raising. Train us to work alongside you in lobbying governments and appearing in the media. Let us help in the office doing whatever we can. Your staff will enjoy meeting us, and we will become a reality to them. Some of us can be passionate advocates for a cure and for support and treatment.

By making us visible, you will be our ally in this struggle to remove the stigma of dementia. You can help us to maintain our identity despite the label of dementia. We can help you to improve services and support.

Help us to discuss issues with our peers, in a safe environment in which we are not judged for our competence. Listen, record, reflect back, capture, summarize and reconstruct our views.

Believe in our potential.
You need us and
we need you.

Run the race for us!

We decline daily. We may not want to or be able to be involved, but we want to be asked.

We need your help.

Be our ally: value us and give us our dignity and individuality.

We need you to run the race towards eliminating stigma for us. DASNI has done, and will do, all it can. But each of us with dementia is declining daily and cannot continue the battle against stigma for very long.

Dudley writes of people labelled with intellectual disability being able to cross the barrier of stigma into the world of 'normals', after a very long struggle with stigma of between ten and 30 years.[4] But people with dementia do not usually have this amount of time to battle stigma.

We could try other options, such as seeking the positives of our disability or pretending to be normal by covering up. But the only viable option for people with dementia, and for the global Alzheimer's movement, is to work together to eliminate the stigma. This will enable society to appreciate the humanity of each person with dementia, at each stage of our increasing disability.

As labelled people, we have the most to gain from eliminating stigma. We must be given the choice to participate in the battle to remove it. Few of us will have the desire or the fortitude to get involved, but we must be given the choice. Self-determination is the key.

Until people with dementia are engaged locally, nationally and internationally, the Alzheimer's movement cannot hear our voice, and cannot develop the services and support for us as consumers.

> Be our ally, value us
> and give us our dignity
> and individuality.

4   James R. Dudley (1997) *Confronting the Stigma in Their Lives*. Springfield, IL: Charles C. Thomas, pp.43–51.

Nothing about us, without us!

Use us as a visible representative of our shared cause.

As we become more visible, the stigma will slowly disappear.

Become our loyal allies, and use people with dementia as visible representatives in the shared cause of eliminating stigma. Don't rely on the stereotype or myth to garner funds. Rely on the real thing – the people with dementia. The stereotype and myth of dementia cannot be sustained when we become seen as individuals. As we become more visible, as our subjective experience is explored, we will be able to influence our quality of life.

Together we can enhance the self-worth of people with dementia, as well as enhance the services and support provided through the global Alzheimer's movement. Together we can challenge the stigma. Let's stand together in the spotlight and adopt the slogan 'Nothing about us, without us!'

7

A bumpy ride

Christine Bryden

June 2010[1]

I was diagnosed with dementia in 1995, at the age of 46. It was a big shock which sent me into depression. My world had changed in the hour in the specialist's rooms. Suddenly, I faced retirement, decline and an unknown future.

Now I am 61, and after all those years I have adapted to a slow but steady decline. Some days, some years, are better than others. Together with friends with dementia that I made online in 2001, we are each making a new life in the slow lane. We feel like survivors of dementia, battling the medical expectations of a rapid decline.

As we age, we feel more in tune with our illness; it seems somehow less inappropriate. Our ageing bodies, with their creaks and groans, now more closely mirror our brain befuddlement.

---

1 Contribution to a Dementia Forum on the Sunshine Coast in June 2010, organized by AA (Sunshine Coast) as part of a wider community Expo on Healthy Lifestyle and Ageing. During this talk, I interviewed Christine (unscripted), in a 'Q&A' style, on her feelings about everyday things – waking up, food, planning, travel, public toilets, shopping malls, pets, sleep, cooking. Audiences appreciated the informal style of the discussion, which helped encourage questions, as well as answering many that were unasked. We often give Q&As.

With Paul alongside me...

I can:

- ▸ live positively
- ▸ advocate for people with dementia
- ▸ do challenging things
- ▸ bounce back
- ▸ conserve my energy and manage stress.

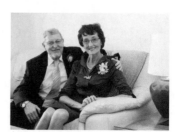

But what have those years since 1995 meant to me and my family?

Without the caring support of my husband, Paul, whom I met three years after diagnosis, I would not have been able to live positively with dementia. He helps where help is needed and steps back to encourage me to keep up skills and to remain bold about my future.

We have travelled so that I could give talks around the world, advocating for more inclusion of and respect for people with dementia. We have moved house, helped our children – doing many things that challenge me. Yet I have also had my bad days, weeks, months and years. By 2006 I was exhausted and wrung out. But this year I am bouncing back, although more cautious about my diminishing energy reserves and sensitivity to stress.

What stresses are there?

I had to:

- redo my will and Power of Attorney
- do two driving assessments
- change to a new neurologist and geriatrician
- find my medical notes.

What are some of the stresses I have experienced?

On moving to Queensland from Canberra, I've had to redo my will and Power of Attorney. Thankfully, I was regarded by my doctor as still being capable of doing this.

I had a few years of driving with medical clearance from my GP, but then had to do two driving assessments with an occupational therapist. This certainly is not for the faint-hearted – driving a strange car, in a strange area, with two strangers, as well as looking at complicated pictures of roads and answering questions.

I've had to change to a new neurologist and then to a new geriatrician, after seven years of ongoing care in Sydney with the neurologist who diagnosed me.

Another stress for me was my GP moving to set up a new practice and taking all my notes (including all those I had transferred from Canberra). After paying to have these sent to me, I am now a supporter of an online system, so that my years of records don't disappear with the doctor.

I no longer feel that I have ongoing GP oversight, as the new practice means I have to wait at least two hours and cannot make an appointment but simply hope to see my regular doctor.

It's a bumpy ride

I am not deaf or stupid but have some trouble communicating.

My memory is uncertain and so annoying.

I get stressed and tired, drifting around needing some direction.

It's a bumpy ride, this journey with dementia.

I have trouble communicating; words fumble around in my head. I am not deaf or stupid; just my communication pathway is scrambled. It all adds to stress and saps my energy. I get tired very easily.

Memory is so uncertain – I open my mouth to say something important, and suddenly it has disappeared in the short trip from my brain to my mouth. Unless I write down a task – even in the middle of the night – it will not get done. So each step of cleaning, cooking, organizing must be written down for me to follow. Otherwise I drift around aimlessly and wonder what I was meant to do.

The stress of coping makes me short-tempered, and the frustration of an unreliable memory simply adds to this.

Maybe now we could pause for a short interview.

Interview

Paul talks to Christine

Background to my journey with dementia for interviewer:

- Age 46, at work, single mum, three girls nine, 13 and 19 when diagnosed and told to retire. Wrote first book, *Who will I be when I die?*[2] (1998). Book title reflects fear of future loss of identity. Diagnosis initially Alzheimer's; changed to probable rare variant of fronto-temporal dementia in 1998.

- 1998, helped to set up support groups in Canberra. Positive outlook, met Paul, married 1999. Started advocacy nationally and internationally with Paul's support.

- 2003, first book translated into Japanese, documentary seen by 10 million. Second book (*Dancing with Dementia*[3]) commissioned by Japanese publisher for release at international conference 2004. Book title reflects daily adaptation to my needs in the form of a dance to the changing music of dementia decline.

- Big change in Japan over next few years – from lack of support for 'demented elderly' and families to lots of community and other support for people with cognitive problems and their families.

- Elected to Board of Alzheimer's Disease International, 2003; stepped down in 2006 when exhausted, burnt out.

- Second book published in UK, 2005; first book translated into Korean and Chinese. Second book translated into Chinese – now to be published in German, 2011.

- Three daughters – three different reactions: over-protective care (eldest), withdrawal into denial (middle one), victim (youngest). Now each one is a wonderful young woman, adjusted to my glacially slow but inevitable decline.

---

2   Christine Bryden (2012) *Who will I be when I die?* London: Jessica Kingsley Publishers (first published 1998).

3   Christine Bryden (2005) *Dancing with Dementia: My Story of Living Positively with Dementia.* London: Jessica Kingsley Publishers.

We are unique human beings

People with dementia each have a story.

Please respect us and value us.

People with dementia should be respected for all that they have contributed during their lives. We each have a story; each one of us is a person of value, of dignity, of worth. Please respect us and value us, despite our difficulty in communicating and understanding.

All that you do to help us makes a tremendous difference to how we cope with increasing difficulties in daily living.

Thank you.

8

The support that I need

Christine Bryden

August 2010[1]

Living with my diagnosis of dementia since 1995 has given me lots of time to think about what care and support I need – what it feels like and what you can do to help. It has been a 15-year journey of slow but steady decline, during which time I have written several articles and two books, as well as given talks and interviews. These efforts were my attempt to advocate for people with dementia: to speak out for all those who cannot or are reluctant to tell you what it feels like and what we need.

Life is becoming increasingly difficult now, but I am still trying to manage my energy and stress levels so that I can give talks like this one.

Thank you so much for inviting me to participate today. It has been very interesting, with really good contributions from a wide range of caring and skilled people. I'll try to leave some time for questions later – for Paul and me – so that you can follow up on what is a necessarily brief insider's perspective of dementia.

---

1   Presentation to a Dementia Symposium arranged by the Western Sydney Dementia Services Alliance (Government and Not-for-Profit Groups) in August 2010, involving professionals and workers, family and people with dementia.

Becoming a labelled person

Problems since 1988.

Medical tests in 1995.

Diagnosed with Alzheimer's disease, then frontal-temporal dementia.

Living in fear and shame.

First, though, how did I become a person labelled with dementia?

I had headaches and confusion, getting lost and stressed since the late 1980s. But all of this I thought was because of my stressful job and personal circumstances. Finally, I had brain scans in 1995 to see why I had headaches, and these showed lots of brain damage, sufficient to diagnose dementia.

The day before my diagnosis I was a busy and successful 46-year-old divorced mother of three girls, with a high-level executive job in the Australian Prime Minister's Department. The day after I was a label – Person with Dementia. No one knew what to say, what to expect of me, how to talk to me and whether even to visit me. I had become a labelled person, defined by my disease overnight. It was as if I had a target painted on my forehead, shouting out for all the world to see that I was blindfolded, no longer able to function in society.

My first two years were a struggle of living a life transformed by this label of dementia. I felt shame and retreated from society. This isolation and depression is often the result of the stigma of having dementia. There was no support for someone with dementia, as it was all directed towards carers. There was no one to talk to about my fears about my future. How would it feel to die with this disease?

My book...

Who am I?

- ‣ Denier
- ‣ Victim
- ‣ Realist

Who will I be when I die?

- ‣ Emotional being
- ‣ Spiritual self

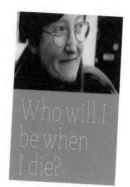

I was encouraged to write about these feelings, and wrote my first book, *Who will I be when I die?*,[2] in the first two years after diagnosis.

My biggest fear was the later stages when I will not know who I am, who my family and friends are, and maybe even not know God. Fear can transform us into **deniers**, when we pretend we are well and nothing is wrong. The fragile shell of normalcy protects us from our fears. And our family and friends deny there is a problem, as a defence against their own feelings of grief and anger. Or fear can paralyze us into becoming a **victim**, giving up our willingness to keep trying to function. And our family and friends adopt the new identity as 'carers', smothering us with their concerns and taking over our daily lives. But we can become a **realist**, reacting to the fears raised by our diagnosis by reflecting on the totality of who we are.

We are far more than a cognitive self. We are emotional beings with relationships in this world with others. We are spiritual selves in relationship with the divine. But we face a medical model of dementia that shapes our fears.

---

2 Christine Bryden (2012) *Who will I be when I die?* London: Jessica Kingsley Publishers (first published 1998).

My 2001 MRI scan

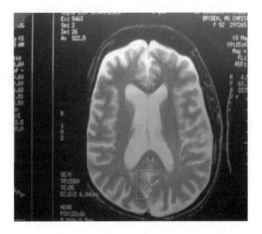

It has been a long journey for me since 1995 to learn how to cast aside my fears and begin to live positively with my diagnosis of dementia.

My scan is a potent symbol of a life transformed into biological inferiority by the medical model of dementia. This early MRI scan, taken in May 2001, shows the relentless progress of destruction of my brain that had already occurred. The medical notes read as follows:

> Cerebral atrophy is present and it is more focal in the frontal and temporal lobes with prominence of the silvian fissures. There is, however, also a degree of central atrophy and atrophy involving the occipital lobes. Cerebellar atrophy is also present... Though the fronto-temporal atrophy is certainly more well established than atrophy elsewhere, it is present elsewhere including a degree of central atrophy.

Later scans – whether SPECT, PET, CAT or MRI[3] (the alphabet soup of radiology!) – simply confirm the earlier medical expectations of steady decline. I seem to have less and less brain each year.

---

3   Single-photon emission computed tomography (SPECT) uses a radioactive trace substance and special camera to create 3-D pictures. A positron emission tomography (PET) scan uses a radioactive trace substance to look at how the body (in this case the brain) functions. Computerized axial tomography (CAT) scans produce cross-sectional images of the body using X-rays. Magnetic resonance imaging (MRI) uses a magnetic field and radio waves to take pictures of the body's interior.

My scan is my curse – a symbol of a life transformed

The 'dementia script': 'You have about five years till you're demented, then about three years till death.'

This is like a hospice in slow motion.

But biology is not the only determinant of function, nor of my humanity.

These scans have been part of the curse of medical prognosis. I was told – like so many others – the standard dementia script: 'You have about five years till you are really demented, then about three years after that in care before you die.' This is like a hospice in slow motion.

But biology is not the sole determinant of my function, nor of my humanity. In what way has this damaged brain made me biologically inferior? In what way am I just a brain and not a whole person?

Haven't I heard about this before? The lepers of earlier days. The Jews in the Holocaust. The blacks under Apartheid? Don't we know that we are all part of a rich tapestry of humanity?

Why are people with dementia still shunned by society, denied respect and dignity, left to retreat in shame? Why do we all believe the dementia script of becoming demented and dying in a certain number of years – despite each of us being unique human beings in very different environments, of differing backgrounds and abilities? And what about the hope of treatment and being cared for with dignity and respect?

Treatment delayed is treatment denied

Drugs at diagnosis slow decline, so do not delay treatment!

I still function OK due to medication, as well as my previous ability.

It's like I used to juggle more balls than most, and can still keep a few in the air!

Why are many of us not offered medication? Often we are just told the 'dementia script' of decline, then death, and given no hope.

At the moment of diagnosis, please give us anti-dementia medication to slow further functional decline. These tablets or skin patches can help what remains to work better, but they do not stop the damage. It is vital to take medication as early as possible. Remember, treatment delayed is treatment denied.

My functioning seems OK because of my Exelon skin patch, without which I could not travel or talk. But it is not only this that helps, but also my previous level of education and ability.

My doctor says it is as if I used to juggle six balls, whereas most people juggle three at most. I have dropped maybe four balls now because of the brain damage, but I still juggle almost as many balls as the ordinary person I meet each day.

Importantly, though, this means I can still speak and tell you what it feels like to have dementia. I still struggle with the decline of this disease, despite an apparent level of remaining function. I can share with you some of my feelings at the early stages of this journey from diagnosis into further decline.

So what does it feel like?

My identity crisis

▸ Who am I?

My environment is vital

▸ Where am I?

My daily struggle

▸ How can I cope?

This journey often begins with thoughts about who we are and who we will become. We face an identity crisis. We have fear of the future, fear of decline, fear of death in a state of unknowing. We can no longer be defined by our work, our contribution to the community, but have a new identity thrust upon us as a diseased person – no longer valued by society, no longer needed for making any contribution.

Help is often directed towards our carers, our friends and families. Suddenly, we have become a non-person. And we are very susceptible to our environment.

- If you do everything for us, we will rapidly forget functions.
- If you don't listen to us, we may give up the struggle to speak.

We face a daily struggle to cope. Each day is filled with a myriad of activities which become more and more difficult as time goes by. Our life becomes fragmented, as each task seems bigger and more overwhelming, so that we lose the interconnectedness of our thread of life.

What's it like?

Existing in the present moment, looking at life unrolling before me and behind me like a carpet.

The diary IS my life, recording all that has happened and will happen in my life.

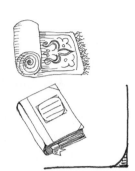

So what is it like?

I talk about this in my second book, which is called *Dancing with Dementia*,[4] drawing on the views of many others with dementia, as well as observations of those in residential care. But in this talk I'll just pick out a few things. I'll start with what it really feels like to have memory problems.

My life is like a carpet unrolling before and behind me. I only know what's happening where I stand at the moment, so that I am totally reliant on my diary. Mostly, if something is not written in the diary, it has not happened or will not happen. Ask me how my day was and I'll have to look at the diary to find out. Tell me you're going out, and in surprise I'll look at the diary and find out where you are going, while also loudly expressing my dismay that something is going to happen that I did not know about – but how could I, if I don't remember?

It's not much use saying to me, 'Wasn't that a lovely day?' I can only express how I feel at the present moment, not how I might have felt at some time during the day, unless you help me to remember what you are talking about.

---

4   Christine Bryden (2005) *Dancing with Dementia: My Story of Living Positively with Dementia*. London: Jessica Kingsley Publishers.

Our environment

Keep it simple:

- encourage routine
- make sure there's only one thing happening at a time.

Understand our aggression or apathy as adaptive behaviour.

We are very susceptible to our environment. Keep it quiet, calm and simple.

My brain finds it very hard to cope. Often I am overwhelmed by different stimuli – music, talking, reading, TV, decisions to make. Then I get really stressed, anxious, tired, exhausted, very frustrated and irritated. I'm glad I can still speak – even if words come out very peculiarly in times like this. At least I can flap my arms around and shout at you.

If you put us in such confusing surroundings, the only other alternative is to withdraw, as it is too difficult to function. Understand this aggression or apathy as *adaptive* – not challenging – behaviour. If you try to speak to me in this sort of environment, I can't follow what you are saying. If I try to speak, words come out mixed up. Half a word or phrase is what I meant to say; the other half will be derived from what I'm hearing around me. It's as if a scrambler is in my brain, mixing up the inputs and outputs. Nor will I be able to concentrate on what you are saying and I will get very confused, so I'll need some quiet time to restore my energy.

Encourage routine so that we can feel safe and secure in a familiar environment, with a set of activities that we can recall. This will reduce the stress of trying to make sense of our surroundings.

Communication

'Listen with your eyes' as we try to tell you how we feel.

Value us so we feel in relationship with you.

It's the way you talk to us, not what you say, that matters.

Just be with us – your caring presence is enough.

We need you to listen carefully as we can't repeat our words. We struggle to speak and it often comes out in a very scrambled way, without proper grammar and syntax. You may be able to help us try to retrieve a memory by finding a word, or a sentence, or a description of the event.

Questions like 'Do you remember?' will make me panic. The black curtain falls down behind me as I desperately try to search for some recollection connecting to what you are asking. Descriptions of your own recollections are much more helpful, as sometimes these trigger my memory so I can share my own feelings with you.

Listen 'with your eyes' – listen to our feelings. This is what we are trying to tell you, even if it makes no sense to you. Sometimes you may need to understand that we just want you to go away – it is too hard to make any type of conversation. But, mostly, the sense of being listened to, being heard, will make us feel valued and in a relationship with you. This is what we need as we cope with shattered thoughts and fragmented selves. It's the way you talk to us, not what you say, that matters. Just be with us – your caring presence is what matters most.

Visiting

It's not a cognitive event but an emotional connection.

It's the way you talk to us, not what you say, that we will remember.

This is what is so important to understand when visiting us.

Please keep visiting us, even if we might not remember that you came before, or even who you are. We may not be able to attach a label to you, but we know your smile and your caring warmth. The emotion of your visit, the friendly feelings you give to us, are far more important than what you say and whether we remember. It is no longer a cognitive event but an emotional connection.

So, as we become more emotional and less cognitive, it's the way you talk to us, not what you say, that we will remember. We know the feeling but don't know the plot. Your smile, your laugh and your touch are what we will connect with.

Encourage our family to keep visiting. Let them know how much they could give us in the way of a positive experience. Of course, if there is tension and conflict, or pain and tears, please remember that this is what we will connect with, even if all the words are pleasant and soothing. We may not recognize them – but is this important if they are giving us a truly pleasant feeling of family warmth and love? It is the emotion we connect to, not the cognitive awareness of the event. This is what is so important to understand when visiting us.

Spirituality

We are losing our cognitive self, even a reliable and coherent emotional self.

What remains is a spiritual self – whatever gave us true meaning in life – that you can connect with.

Make sure you know what that was, before connecting with us – it's not a time for conversion, but of reminiscence and reflection.

Our faith, or our spirituality, is crucial. We are losing our cognitive self – even a reliable and coherent emotional self. What remains is our spirituality. We need you to help us connect with this, with whatever has given us true meaning in life in the past.

Our emotions have become increasingly scrambled – from apathy to extremes of anger or frustration. Beneath, though, lies our largely intact spiritual self. Even in the very end stages of this journey with dementia, people have shown an awareness of familiar places, music and words from their own faith tradition.

But make sure you know what a person's faith or belief system was, before connecting with us on this level. It's not a time for conversion, but one of reminiscence and reflection. So maybe you help someone to visit church, temple, synagogue, art gallery, gardens – whatever you discover lay at the heart of the person's sense of meaning and purpose in previous years.

In addition to this spiritual core relating to meaning and place, the love of family and friends can give us security, an oasis of emotional warmth in an otherwise confusing world. You are our care-partners on this journey, and we need you to understand us, and to meet our needs as we become less and less able to deal with this illness.

The empathy from our family, friends and even professional carers supports us on this journey into increasing chaos and confusion. You provide an anchor for us to connect with, to hold on to in our time of need.

Keeping an open mind

At diagnosis:

- living with memory loss.

At home alone:

- systems.

At home with family:

- support, education, 'time out'.

Residential care:

- person-centred care
- atmosphere more important than décor.

We need to keep an open mind as to what care and support we need, as this will depend on where we are on this journey from diagnosis to death, and whether we are at home or in care.

At diagnosis we need information, support groups, and perhaps also counselling. At home alone, for example, it's no use asking if I have taken my tablets, as it feels as if I have just done so – or was that yesterday or the day before? So we will need lots of support systems to help us take our tablets, have showers, eat, shop, as well as decide about driving, Powers of Attorney and finding ongoing medical care.

When our families are supporting us, they will themselves need support and education, as well as 'time out'. They need to be able to really understand what it feels like for us, so that they provide routine, and have a fixed place for everything to be kept, as well as bucket loads of patience for our adaptive behaviour.

In residential care, call us by name and remember who we are as a person. Use touch and smiles to connect with us. The care atmosphere of a home is far more important than its decor. Looks can be deceiving. Where Paul and I visit each week, the Eden Alternative[5] is used, and residents are respected as people of value and worth, even though staff are clearly very busy.

> Open your mind – see us as people first and foremost.

---

5 The Eden Alternative® is an international, non-profit organization dedicated to creating quality of life for 'Elders' and their care partners, wherever they may live. Active in the UK, USA, Canada, Australia, New Zealand, Denmark, Austria, Netherlands, South Africa and Faroe Islands.

Where to now?

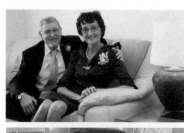

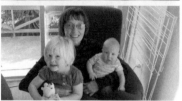

Use it or lose it!

Have a positive attitude.

Live each day to the full.

I have been so blessed to decline much more slowly than expected given the degree of brain damage already apparent on scans in 1995. The neurologist is amazed at the level of function, despite the ongoing damage and declining cognitive ability on testing. But that's the medical model. I prefer a view of 'use it or lose it' and having a positive attitude. As a team with Paul, we can do what is important, not simply urgent, and not get too exhausted in the process. I still advocate for people with dementia, but not as often. We still travel, but less frequently and in a less frenetic way.

Our youngest daughter is on track for an academic career. Last year (2009) our middle daughter was married and here we are dressed up ready for the event. And we have two delightful grandchildren from my eldest daughter – as you can see! I never thought it possible that I would live long enough to see all of this. The trauma to my family as a divorced mum of three daughters in the few years after diagnosis seems now so long ago. Only echoes of that time remain, far outweighed by the delights of this new life in the slow lane.

So where to now? I shall give talks, keep the website updated, travel as and when I can, and continue to visit our local nursing home. Who knows what lies ahead for any of us, but I plan to make the most of my life as it unrolls before me like a carpet full of surprises.

Thank you for inviting me to share in this event with you.

9

Stigma and fear

Christine Bryden

March 2011[1]

I have lived now with a diagnosis of dementia for 16 years, beating any projections made by the doctors. I have battled the physical symptoms of this disease and coped with lots of ups and downs.

When I was diagnosed, the society and medical view of dementia was one of despair, there being nothing to do except go home and prepare to die, and to wither away in the mind until I was an empty shell. My talk is about how I cast aside the stigma put upon me by society, and tackled the fear within for my future.

I became an active advocate for people with dementia, first speaking within Australia. My first talk outside of my home country was at Murray Alzheimer Research and Education Program in mid-2001! And here I am a decade later, still here and still talking.

> My message today is that
> you can live positively with
> dementia and enjoy each
> new day in the slow lane.

---

1 Presentation to the Murray Alzheimer's Research and Education Program (University of Waterloo, Canada), immediately preceding (at the same venue) the 26th ADI Conference in Toronto in March 2011.

What causes stigma and fear?

The stereotype of dementia leads to:

▸ stigma in society, and

▸ fear in the person diagnosed.

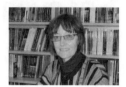

What is the cause of the stigma and fear? It's the **stereotype** of dementia: someone who cannot understand, remembers nothing and is unaware of what is happening around them. This stereotype **tugs at the heartstrings and loosens the purse strings**, so is used in seeking funds for research, support and services. It's a Catch 22, because Alzheimer's associations promote our image as non-persons and make the stigma worse.

Stigma is a disease of society resulting from the stereotype. We are shunned by former work colleagues, and our friends become awkward in our presence, with the picture of a non-person – the stereotype of the empty shell – clouding their perception of us. Stigma becomes an invisible veil of misunderstanding, masking our potential and segregating us from normal society.

Fear is what matters most to the person being diagnosed. We fear becoming the empty shell – the non-person – portrayed in the stereotype. Our fear is a basic survival mechanism in response to the threat of future danger – of death in this state of non-being. Fear can be paralyzing.

What causes stigma and fear?

Frankl: need to find meaning in life to combat the 'trauma of non-being'.

At diagnosis we fear a state of non-being, even before death arrives to release us.

According to Viktor Frankl, author of *Man's Search for Meaning*,[2] when a person is faced with death, the most basic of all human wishes is to find a meaning in life to combat the 'trauma of non-being'.

Misunderstanding and stigma have significant implications for those of us diagnosed with dementia. We face the trauma of non-being, even before death arrives to release us.

How can we face this fear?

---

2   Viktor E. Frankl (1985) *Man's Search for Meaning.* New York: Washington Square Press.

How did I overcome my fear?

Depression till met Liz in 1996, then two years of journeying together.
Encouraged to write about my feelings.

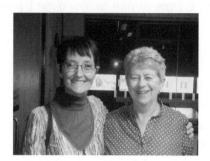

How did I face my fears and find a sense of meaning in life? I was diagnosed in May 1995 and became depressed and fearful, until I met a wonderful friend in 1996, in whom I could confide.

Each month I would meet with Liz MacKinlay, a theologian, priest and geriatric nurse and professor. We both had to challenge the stereotype, address society's stigma and tackle the fear that was paralyzing me. Together we went on a journey of discovery. Liz encouraged me to write a book about my experiences, so I could help change the stereotype. This gave me my sense of meaning in life: to speak out for all those being diagnosed, to encourage others and to advocate for better support and services, as well as recognition and inclusion.

By 'coming out' openly as a person with dementia, by talking in the media and in my book about what it feels like, I was directly challenging the stereotype. How could I be an empty shell if I could still talk? But also, if I could talk, did I really have dementia? So I was ignoring the stigma in order to tackle my fear.

How did I overcome my fear?

'He who conceals his disease cannot expect to overcome it.'

For me, talking, writing and sharing have helped a great deal in addressing my fear. Like the Ethiopian proverb: 'He who conceals his disease cannot expect to overcome it.' If I had concealed my fear or, even worse, given in to it, I could have rapidly been on a downward spiral into depression.

If we accept the label of dementia and the stigma of the stereotype, we fear each loss; we fear a decline into the expected behaviours of dementia. We assume that we will become the empty shell. Isolated by stigma, we are left alone with our fear, of decline into a state of non-being, followed by death. But it doesn't have to be that way. We can live a new life in the slow lane of dementia, with the support of others who understand.

Tackling fear head on

Swindoll: 'I'm convinced that life is 10% what actually happens to me, and 90% how I react to it.'

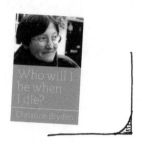

With Liz's encouragement, I wrote my first book.[3] Its title expresses the fear so many of us have at diagnosis. Who will we be when we die? Will we be an empty shell? Liz reassured me that I would retain my spiritual self, and set my fears in the bedrock of faith and hope. My Christian faith gives me my sense of meaning and of hope.

My motto, as Charles Swindoll is quoted as saying, was: 'I'm convinced that life is 10% what actually happens to me, and 90% how I react to it'. I realized there was much I could still do, while also accepting the possibility of decline.

---

3 Christine Bryden (2012) *Who will I be when I die?* London: Jessica Kingsley Publishers (first published 1998).

Tackling fear head on!

Nietzsche: 'He who has a why to live for can bear with almost any how.'[4]

Monty Python: 'Always look on the bright side of life.'

Addressing stigma and fear in my life meant:

- Finding a sense of meaning in my life. Nietzsche said that he who has a *why* to live can bear with almost any *how*.

- Focusing on personal relationships based on love and connectedness. We then have people alongside us to help provide calm in the storms of anxiety and frustration.

- Looking for the positives – 'Always look on the bright side of life' (*Monty Python's Life of Brian*) – and of course finding humour in the absurdity of life.

My past way of being bold and challenging accepted norms of behaviour reasserted itself. By early 1998 I had ignored the stigma and refused to succumb to fear. Others might call this denial or lack of acceptance. I started (and later completed) a graduate diploma in pastoral care and counselling – not usually recommended for those with dementia. But then it was my next act that was to really alarm my daughters, who thought I was now showing all the signs of losing it!

---

4   Friedrich Nietzsche, quoted by Viktor E. Frankl (1985) *Man's Search for Meaning*. New York: Washington Square Press.

Care-partners

Boden became Bryden, and much more than a few letters changed!

Paul and I became care-partners in the dance of dementia.

Now I had a personal relationship based on love and connectedness.

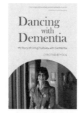 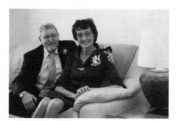

I signed up to a dating agency and met a lovely man, Paul, and married him a year later. Boden became Bryden. By changing a few letters of my name, far more had changed!

Paul became my support, my care-partner in this dance to the changing melody of dementia. I now had a personal relationship based on love and connectedness. I had him alongside me to help provide calm in the storms of anxiety and frustration.

I wrote a second book about what it feels like to have dementia and what you can do to help.[5] It was also a story of my amazing journey with dementia, meeting and marrying Paul, and experiencing this roller-coaster ride of ups and downs. The changing music of dementia meant we needed to adapt our care-partnership, but it also gave us much to be thankful for and much to share.

But although I had overcome my fear by not accepting the stereotype, still I was isolated by the stigma of society. Like a web, the stigma that arises from the stereotype traps us in a medical dementia system. Alone, I could not change society. But, with Paul's help, I felt empowered to work with others for change.

---

5   Christine Bryden (2005) *Dancing with Dementia: My Story of Living Positively with Dementia.* London: Jessica Kingsley Publishers.

The ultimate in boldness!

2001: DASNI formed and challenged the stereotype.

We approached ADI seeking change and were taken seriously.

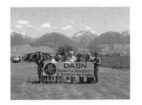

We also changed – no longer limited by our own fears.

The DASNI effect emboldened us.

Many of those who met in Montana in 2001 are still here and active in advocacy!

In late 2000 I joined an internet group of others with dementia. In 2001 we met in Montana, flying the banner of advocacy and change, forming the Dementia Advocacy and Support Network International (DASNI). We gave each other new hope simply by being ourselves. Together we started to work to change the stereotype and so reduce the stigma of dementia.

We approached Alzheimer's Disease International (ADI), seeking inclusion and improved services and support. In so doing, we were challenging the stereotype of how a person with dementia should behave. We argued for acceptance as valued human beings, not simply those labelled with dementia.

We needed to act together to challenge the stereotype. As a group we could not be written off as individual freaks who did not really have dementia because we could speak. We were taken seriously. There was change in how they included us and sought our input.

Importantly, we also changed. No longer limited by our own fears, the DASNI effect emboldened us. Many of the people who met in Montana in 2001 are still here and active in advocacy! One of the changes that ADI made had a big impact on me.

2002–2010

Elected to ADI Board 2003 and active member until ADI Berlin 2006.

Active advocacy in Japan from 2002 to 2007.

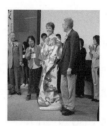

In 2003 I was elected to ADI's Governing Board, which was a great honour, and yet a daunting prospect of travel to meetings and networking on issues papers. I tried my best to represent the interests of all those with dementia, whether they could express themselves or not.

At the same time I had become very active in advocacy in Japan. I worked with a network of media, care-providers and government ministries to prepare for major change. In 2004 Japan hosted the international Alzheimer's Disease International conference in Kyoto, and was referring to people with dementia as the 'demented elderly'. Within two years that had changed to 'people with cognitive problems'. Now Japanese people with dementia are speaking openly about their needs, are being heard, and their needs are being met.

2002–2010

But burn-out, stress, anxiety, losing sleep and weight.

Maybe the sun was finally setting on my journey of dementia.

I focused inwards on family, gardening, reading.

But at home I was experiencing burn-out, losing sleep and weight, struggling with a rising tide of anxiety and stress. Now maybe my fears were being realized, and the confusion of dementia was becoming too much for me? I stepped down from ADI's Board in 2006, and struggled even to meet my remaining commitments in Japan till 2007.

I focused on our family. The delights of our daughter's wedding and of grandchildren, born in 2007 and 2010, were highlights in an otherwise restricted and more gloomy outlook. These mileposts were not ones I thought I would reach when diagnosed in 1995. Now they were reached, would I now decline further into the empty shell? Would I finally succumb to the stereotype of dementia?

2011 onwards!

Meeting old friends at ADI
Thessaloniki March 2010.

Talk in Sydney July 2010.

Back on the journey of advocacy.

Casting aside fear again!

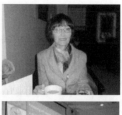
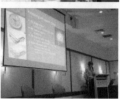

Far from it! Paul persuaded me to go to ADI's conference in Thessaloniki last March where I met old friends and felt energized once more. Soon I was responding positively to requests to give talks, such as the one in Sydney last July, called 'The support that I need.'[6] I had a website developed and felt much encouraged by the emails arriving from people around the world who had read my books and heard my talks.

My health was still a battle, but I began to have some insight into my problems, which all seemed to trace back to very high levels of anxiety. Not being aware of time, nor of the past or future, life in this limbo-land of dementia can be a very stressful place. So, with the help of calmatives, I was able to cast aside the fear of decline yet again and to cope better with daily life. And even travelling and speaking once more!

---

6   See Chapter 8.

I'm still here!

Your life has meaning, treasure this!

Find a friend – focus on relationships based on love and connectedness.

Look for positives and humour in the absurdity of life.

Find a group who knows what it feels like and supports you.

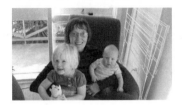

So now I am still here and want to do all I can while I can to help change the stereotype of dementia. It is this picture of the state of non-being that leads to the stigma of society and isolates us in our fear of becoming this empty shell. The journey with dementia certainly has its challenges, but it also has its joys and, in the face of stigma, we often forget that.

If you are living with dementia like I am, don't let fear mask the worth you still have and always will have. **Know that your life has meaning** and nurture this sense of meaning in your life. **Find a friend who will listen and encourage** and look for relationships based on love and connectedness. **Look for the positives in life** and discover the humour that exists in the absurdity of life. And **find a group who knows what it feels like and will support you** – even take action with you. For me this is DASNI, but it also may be an early-stage support group or other group.

Working together, we can prevent stigma and fear.

It is possible, it is achievable, today not tomorrow!

If I can speak, I can still have dementia. If I can speak, I can tell you what it feels like and what you can do to help. Listen! Reach out over the barrier of stigma and help us overcome our fears. If we work together, we can prevent stigma and fear. It is possible, it is achievable, today not tomorrow.

Thank you.

NOTHING ABOUT US, WITHOUT US!

10

I'm still here!

Christine Bryden

March 2011[1]

I was the first person with dementia to give a plenary address to an ADI conference, ten years ago. Paul reminded me that it was in Christchurch, where there has been that dreadful earthquake. So many have died, so much has been damaged, including the Hotel Grand Chancellor where some of us stayed. My talk back then was called 'Diagnosis, drugs and determination'.[2] Since 2001, by taking anti-dementia drugs and tackling my fear with determination, I'm still here!

In this talk I reflect on the past decade of change: in my own personal journey, for an amazing group of people with dementia, and the response of ADI and its members.

So, when did it all start?

---

1   Opening Plenary address to the 26th ADI Conference in Toronto, March 2011. Christine reviewed the positive changes that had occurred in attitudes towards dementia over the ten years since she was the first person with a diagnosis to address ADI, and what further progress was needed.

2   See Chapter 2.

The first steps…

Paralyzed by fear that 'things are in the unmaking'.

▸ Wrote book about fear –
  Who will I be when I die?

Free 'to choose one's attitude'.

▸ Met and married Paul.

▸ Together we could steer through the troubled waters of dementia!

With his support, there was much I could do!

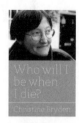

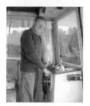

In 1995, with my diagnosis at the age of only 46. I faced the terror of becoming the stereotype of dementia which is of an empty shell. As American author Stephen King says: 'Terror…arises from a pervasive sense of disestablishment; that things are in the unmaking.'[3] I faced my own 'unmaking' and became paralyzed by fear. But a friend encouraged me to write about this and my first book emerged, titled *Who will I be when I die?*[4]

After a year or so of depression, I chose to be positive and challenge the stereotype of dementia. Concentration camp survivor Viktor Frankl said: 'Everything can be taken from man but one thing: the last of human freedoms – to choose one's attitude in any given set of circumstances.'[5]

I certainly challenged the stereotype when I went to an introductions agency and met Paul. Married in 1999, together we could steer through the troubled waters of dementia. With his support, I could do so much more. I began to talk about what it feels like to have dementia.

A decade ago I spoke at the Australian Alzheimer's Association national conference. This led to so much more speaking out!

---

3   Stephen King (2010) *Danse Macabre*. New York: Gallery Books (first published 1981), p.8.

4   Christine Bryden (2012) *Who will I be when I die?* London: Jessica Kingsley Publishers (first published 1998).

5   Viktor E. Frankl (1985) *Man's Search for Meaning*. New York: Washington Square Press, p.86.

Ten-year roller-coaster ride!

2001 NZ plenary address.

2003 Talks around world.

2003 Elected to ADI Board.

2003 Started to focus on Japan.

2007 Retreated to delight of family.

2010 Inspired by ADI friends in Greece.

'What doesn't destroy me makes me stronger.'

Famous people hold out the beacon of hope for creative suffering!

It's not all downhill!

I was invited to give the plenary address for ADI in New Zealand. Friends with dementia from other countries were there, making a big impact on delegates, many of whom had never spoken to a person with dementia. We were not empty shells!

In 2003 I went round the world to speak at conferences of ADI and its members, then focusing more on Japan in the lead-up to ADI in Kyoto in 2004. But by 2007 I struggled to meet remaining commitments and retreated from advocacy. Although there were family events I never thought I would live to see, such as a wedding and grandchildren, my health was a battleground. Mysterious stomach ailments led to loss of weight, then being unable to walk due to knee and foot pain. I declined into exhaustion and confusion. When Paul suggested we go to ADI at Thessaloniki, I didn't want to go, but once there, among old friends, I felt invigorated.

So my roller-coaster ride has not been all downhill! The black American activist Martin Luther King said: 'What doesn't destroy me makes me stronger.'[6] Like other famous people, he holds out the beacon of hope for creative suffering.

But what have these years with dementia felt like?

---

6   Phillip Yancey (1990) *Where Is God When It Hurts?* Grand Rapids, MI: Zondervan, p.144.

Kaleidoscope of past and present

Without a future, resulting in anxiety and panic:

- past is cloud shifting to reveal memory
- present is jagged, flickering fragments
- future blank sheet full of surprises.

Life became dominated by mania and panic:

- had insight and took calmatives.

Yet there are blissful moments of clarity with bursts of normality breaking through the fog!

It's been a kaleidoscope of past and present, without a future. The past is a shifting cloud, occasionally lifting to show a memory. The present is jagged flickering fragments, and the future is a blank sheet full of surprises. Both past and future are reconstructed in discussion with Paul, but I rely on his description, so my own reality is lost.

Unless I write things down, and find the note, each day is full of shocks, as I don't know what we've planned. We're off tomorrow – where? How was your friend yesterday – who? Today's fun – why? So many questions with no answers! So there are half-done tasks, and an exhausting focus on what I'm doing right now, to the exclusion of whatever else I might have meant to do.

In 2004, in the midst of this manic struggle, I wrote my second book, describing what it feels like and what you can do to help.[7] The title, *Dancing with Dementia*, is a metaphor for the way Paul and I have adapted to the changing tune of dementia.

By last year, my life was dominated by anxiety and panic, so extreme to the point of nausea and vomiting. But then I had a rare moment of insight and talked to my doctor, who gave me calmatives. Now life is less stressful, but still tiring. Without Paul's support, I could not live at home. I would forget to eat, place myself in danger, and decline without regular medication.

So this dance with dementia has its downside, but it also has bursts of normality breaking through the fog of confusion. I'm still here and so are others.

What does this say to us?

---

7 Christine Bryden (2005) *Dancing with Dementia: My Story of Living Positively with Dementia*. London: Jessica Kingsley Publishers.

NOTHING ABOUT US, WITHOUT US!

DASNI made a difference

'It is by those who have suffered that the world has been advanced.'

'Alone we can do so little; together we can do so much.'

'Never doubt that a small group of thoughtful, committed citizens can change the world.'

 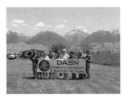

It says people with dementia can survive and thrive, and can make a difference. As Russian author Leo Tolstoy has said: 'It is by those who have suffered that the world has been advanced.'[8]

In 2001, by gathering together as a group of people with dementia among the mountains of Montana, the Dementia Advocacy and Support Network International (DASNI) raised a banner for change, and over the next two years worked with ADI, seeking recognition and inclusion, and to be full participants in all of ADI activities.

Our symbol is the turtle because we are slower than we used to be, but it has wings to show how we can rise and cover the globe. The forget-me-not flower signifies our wish to be remembered. Our collective strengths enable us to participate and achieve. As Helen Keller said: 'Alone we can do so little; together we can do so much.'[9]

---

8   *The Vegetarian*, London newspaper of The International Vegetarian Union, December 21 1889.

9   American Helen Keller (1880–1968) was born blind and deaf, and learned to speak, becoming a powerful advocate for disabled people. These words are from Dorothy Herrmann (1998) *Helen Keller: A Life.* Chicago: University of Chicago Press, p.222.

All but one of these remarkable DASNI heroes, who made such an impact on ADI, are still active. Three of us are here today: Lynn Jackson, Jan Phillips and me. These DASNI heroes are featured in the booklet in your delegates' bag, which makes for inspiring reading. These words, often attributed to Margaret Mead, the US anthropologist, say it so well: 'Never doubt that a small group of thoughtful, committed citizens can change the world.'

People with dementia are not freaks, but experts on what it feels like to have dementia. We can reach out to the world that we have left behind on this journey with dementia.

But how have we been able to survive and thrive?

The DASNI effect – Client Survival Initiative

- Surviving and thriving.
- Proactive in advocating for social justice.
- Active supporters of each other through 3300 messages and 15,000 hours of chat.
- DASNI effects shows it to be a CSI, not crime scene investigation of TV series but Client Survival Initiative.

As clients of dementia research, services and support, we claim equal status with you as care-partners for all those with dementia.

We call it the DASNI effect. By being proactive in seeking social justice, we experienced a strong rehabilitative effect. We were not just passive participants in support groups, but active supporters of each other. More than 3300 messages and 15,000 hours of chat over the last decade have reached several hundred otherwise isolated people with dementia.

Back in 2001, we didn't anticipate how great the DASNI effect would be and that many of us would still be functioning at a high level today. We did not know DASNI would become an effective CSI – not the crime scene investigation of the American TV series, but a Client Survivor Initiative. As clients of dementia research, services and support, we claim equal status with you as expert care-partners for all those with dementia.

We now know that CSIs help with social support, empowerment, wellbeing and quality of life. As a CSI, DASNI has provided a safe welcoming place for people with dementia to share with peers, to participate and contribute, and to connect with and make a difference to the research, services and support providers such as ADI and its members.

As survivors, we might make you feel uncomfortable. We do not fit the stereotype, but why is this?

The prison of dementia

Courage to reject label of dementia.

But reality of dementia imprisons us.

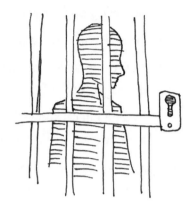

- We don't know how long till it gets worse; it can't get better.

- 'Our inner life changes – we no longer live for the future, aiming for a goal. We remain in limbo, removed from normal life.'

It's a continuing battle against rushing torrent of dementia:

- ongoing neuroplasticity.

It's because we have cast aside the belief in the medical model that imprisoned us. We had the courage to reject the label of dementia that said we had so many years till we became an empty shell. We are still fully human, with our dignity intact. But we remain in the prison of the reality of dementia. We don't know how long till it gets worse; we only know it can't get better.

For some, it's not a question of attitude or brain exercise, as they can't rise above the rushing torrent of dementia. The disease is simply too fast and too relentless. For others, such as the DASNI heroes in your booklet, we survive and thrive despite a continuing battle against continuing loss.

In 2007, though, we were encouraged by the release of the book *The Brain that Changes Itself*.[10] What we knew instinctively – and had experienced as the DASNI effect – was now being given a name: neuroplasticity. We had been able to maintain a lot of function through our own efforts.

But could we recover all lost function?

---

10 Doidge, N. (2007) *The Brain that Changes Itself: Stories of Personal Triumph from the Frontiers of Brain Science.* New York: Viking Penguin.

Up the escalator coming down!

Running up, still slipping back down.

We keep firing, we keep wiring, but we also keep unwiring!

We're hanging on much longer than expected, and have handed the baton to other experts coming after.

'Nothing about us, without us!'

Our story of survival can inspire others being diagnosed today.

Sadly, no. However much we struggle, it's a case of one or two steps forward, then three steps back. But this is better than three steps back each time. We are forming new neural connections by our mental, emotional and physical activity, but these disintegrate with the continuing onslaught of the disease process. As we keep firing, we keep wiring, but we also keep unwiring! Unlike age-related memory loss, where brain exercise can give some hope of recovery, our disease-related dementia requires more effort, more exercise, and acceptance of decline nonetheless.

With support of others, such as in DASNI, we can overcome the hopelessness we might feel. We're hanging on longer than expected and hope our story of survival can inspire others.

We spoke out in 2004 about the need for nothing about us, without us. Back then we said we were handing on the baton of this race to tell you what it feels like, to those coming after us. I have now lasted long enough to reflect on the changes I have seen in ADI and its member countries in response to the approach by DASNI ten years ago. What have I seen in that time?

ADI – the last decade

Much has changed!

From an empty shell, we now have full participation.

I've met people with dementia from around the world in the quiet room.

We're speaking out and being listened to.

We're included in governance and advisory capacities.

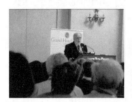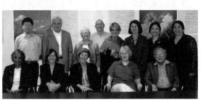

By 2002 ADI had revised its Charter of Principles and produced a factsheet about recognition and inclusion of people with dementia. The ADI newsletter often contains our contributions. We are encouraged to attend and to speak at conferences, through sponsorship and concessional registration. In the quiet room, I've met people from Canada, the UK, the USA, Japan, Germany, Macedonia, Singapore and Malaysia.

In 2002 Peter Ashley (pictured) was the second person with dementia to address an ADI conference. By 2003 we were part of ADI governance, with Lynda Hogg from Scotland now on the ADI Board (pictured in the front row, second from the right). Our views are being respected and listened to. ADI is leading many of its members by example. Among ADI member countries there has also been much change. We are involved in media and government liaison to seek more research and improved services and support. And there are other excellent initiatives, such as sections of websites for people who have dementia, and the Scottish Dementia Working Group. But I will now turn to one ADI member as an example of change in a short period of time.

Creating a dementia-friendly society!

From 'demented elderly' to 'people with cognitive deficits'.

Kyoto 2004: Mr Ochi spoke in public to around 4000 people.

Government ten-year plan.

One million trained supporters.

Network of people with dementia.

Meeting in March 2011.

Maybe DASNI Japan?

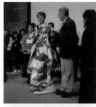

Japan has achieved so much since I first visited in 2003. I gave talks, such as in Matsue where I was given this amazing wedding kimono, and was interviewed for a TV program that reached 10 million viewers. A small group of researchers, day centre workers, government advisors and media were organizing all of this. By the following year, the Japanese publisher of my first book wanted another one in time for ADI Kyoto 2004.

Here Mr Ochi gave the closing plenary address to an audience of around 4000. As the first Japanese person with dementia to speak out, he had a huge impact! The government has since announced a ten-year plan for creating a dementia-friendly society, with one million trained supporters. Instead of the 'demented elderly', we have become people with cognitive deficits.

By 2006, in Kyoto again, a group of people with dementia (pictured) invited me to be present when they drew up a manifesto of what they wanted from government. The next year there was a summit for people with early-onset dementia in Hiroshima.

In the last two years, as part of a developing network, people with dementia have attended more than 150 regional meetings, some including a press conference. Just a few weeks ago there was a national seminar in Osaka for people with dementia, at which I was present through the marvels of Skype. There is now talk of setting up DASNI Japan. What a remarkable change in just a few years!

One Japanese example is truly inspirational!

Restoring identity!

Sapporo music band

Business cards

Music

Fun

Travel

Publicity

People with dementia reclaimed their role in society, with dignity and respect

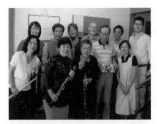

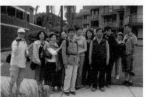

A manager of a day centre in Sapporo has created a music band, including herself, two people with dementia and their wives. Each band member has a business card, which is so important! For a person whose life is their work, their business card represents who they are. After diagnosis, all this changes. But now, for these band members, identity has been restored and respect regained!

We first met the music band, of clarinets and flutes, and visited their day centre in 2007 (pictured). Then they came to Australia in 2008, with a small team of observers. The band gave several recitals to our Association, each of which was a memorable and moving occasion, and is still talked about. An NHK TV crew has followed the band activities and made a documentary that was seen by millions of viewers in Japan.

The amazing change in Japan has been the result of the efforts of many people working together: government ministries, media outlets, professional care-givers and, most importantly, the people with dementia themselves. It is they who have had the most impact. It is through their own activities, their own words and actions, that people with dementia have reclaimed a role in society, with dignity and respect. I feel very honoured to have played a small role as a catalyst in this.

With such examples of change, where do we go from here?

Time is running out!

Let's make dementia a global health priority to address the global health crisis.

Let's 'go forward together with our united strength' and:

- find cures for diseases causing dementia
- improve access to medication
- improve services and support
- create a dementia-friendly society.

Let's dream of a world free from all the diseases that result in dementia.

'With this faith we will be able to hew out of the mountain of despair a stone of hope.'

Time is running out! There is much still to do in developing countries. Diagnosis takes place much later, and there is little access to medication, nor much in the way of services and support.

Over the next decade, more people in both the developing and developed world will be diagnosed and, without cures for the various diseases that cause dementia, we face a global dementia crisis.

Today around the globe there are around 35.6 million people living with dementia. Without cures, this number will dramatically increase, and the cost of care-giving and the impact on families and societies around the world will soar. We must work together to make dementia a global health priority.

As the UK war-time prime minister Winston Churchill said: 'Come then, let us go forward together with our united strength.'[11] Together let's work to find cures, let's improve access to anti-dementia medication, and let's improve services and support to people with dementia and their families.

Let's create a dementia-friendly society. In the next decade, let's dream of one day seeing a world free from all the diseases that result in dementia.

---

11   From Churchill's first speech as Prime Minister to the House of Commons on 13 May 1940. The speech is available at www.winstonchurchill.org/resources/speeches/1940-the-finest-hour/blood-toil-tears-and-sweat, accessed on 2 July 2015.

We people with dementia, and all of you who support us, have achieved so much in just one decade. Let's take Martin Luther King's words to heart: 'With this faith we will be able to hew out of the mountain of despair a stone of hope.'[12]

Thank you.

---

12 Martin Luther King, Jr, 'I Have a Dream', delivered 28 August 1963, at the Lincoln Memorial, Washington D.C.

NOTHING ABOUT US, WITHOUT US!

11

Coming out of the shadow

Christine Bryden

April 2011[1]

I'm Christine Bryden. I was diagnosed with dementia in 1995, at the age of 46. Now 62, I have survived a 16-year journey with dementia. In that time of slow but steady decline, I have spoken to conferences and appeared in the media around the world and written two books. My goal has been to try to describe what it feels like to have dementia and what you can do to help. But, most importantly, I have been a passionate advocate for the rights of people with dementia to participate, to speak out, to come out of the shadow and be part of the community.

So how did I find the courage to speak out and be listened to, back in 2001, when I gave a plenary address to the Alzheimer's Disease International conference – the first by a person with dementia?

---

1   Presentation to events launching the German edition of *Dancing with Dementia* in Zurich and Frankfurt, April 2011.

2001 – DASNI approaches ADI

2001 Dementia Advocacy and Support Network International (DASNI) approached Alzheimer's Disease International (ADI).

Now, people with dementia are writing and speaking at conferences.

Services and support are improving.

People with dementia are being respected as human beings worthy of respect and dignity.

Together we made a difference!

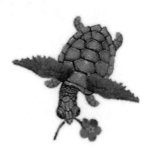

I had found friends on the internet who, like me, had a diagnosis of dementia and wanted to take action, to make a difference. Together we founded Dementia Advocacy and Support Network International (DASNI) in 2001.

We approached Alzheimer's Disease International, asking for their encouragement in coming out of the shadow. Since then so much has changed. People with dementia have spoken at their conferences, and we are being listened to. Services and support are improving in ADI member countries, and people with dementia are being respected as human beings worthy of respect and dignity. Together DASNI did make a difference.

This logo for DASNI symbolizes how we may be as slow as the turtle in our cognition, but the wings show how we can rise and cover the globe with our individual and collective strengths. The forget-me-not flower reminds us of our shared experience, of memory loss and our wish not to be forgotten.

But surely if people with dementia were speaking out, they could not really have dementia? Surely we should fit the stereotype quoted in the 2001 ADI Annual Report: 'the mind is absent and the body is an empty shell'?

Far more than the label of dementia!

Unique psychic resources to draw on coping with brain damage, especially at diagnosis.

Challenging the lies surrounding dementia by living positively with dementia.

With early diagnosis and treatment, we people with dementia function at a higher level.

Finding others to laugh with over our common frailties, share our despair and encourage each other with helpful tips.

But we are far more than brains. We each have a unique personality with emotions, experiences and a place in a social world. We have drawn on our own psychic resources to cope with our brain damage and the difficulties we are experiencing in our daily lives. Most importantly, we needed these resources at the moment of diagnosis.

At first I reacted to the trauma of diagnosis by believing the lie of dementia – that I would decline and there was no hope. I was able to cast this lie aside and challenge accepted wisdom. I fought off depression, to live for today and tomorrow with dignity and cheerfulness. Like my friends in DASNI, I can look to a half-full glass of living positively with dementia.

The half-empty glass of dementia's past developed in the framework of diagnosis only after years of memory loss and confusion, without anti-dementia drugs and with no support groups – face to face or on the internet – in which we could encourage each other.

With earlier diagnosis and early treatment, we people with dementia can function at a far higher level than ever thought possible before. We can find others like ourselves who we can laugh with over our common frailties, share our despair and encourage each other with helpful tips.

But where does this journey start? What are the first signs?

Rumblings of catastrophe…

Allowing others to take over, we risk learned helplessness, but we must 'use it or lose it'!

Toxic power of 'bone-pointing' moment of diagnosis, with terror and dread of downhill decline into 'empty shell'.

Day before diagnosis I was respected; the day after I had become a label: dementia.

From then on, would I only ever be allowed to function with my 'carer' in attendance?

Often the first signs are seen at times of stress. Our world begins to fall apart, as we sense the rumblings of catastrophe. We increasingly use avoidance, and allow others – usually our family – to take over our functioning, often to the stage where we 'forget' how to do it ourselves. We risk losing everything by learned helplessness, forgetting the maxim 'Use it or lose it'.

Then we face the toxic power of the moment of diagnosis. Like the curse of pointing the bone, we believe the medical diagnosis and prognosis. Belief of a downhill decline into an empty shell becomes a self-fulfilling prophecy! We experience terror and dread, when it seems as if our world has come to an end. We fear further loss, and dread what the future holds.

I did not know what function I would lose next, and each mistake became a sign of irreversible decline. I was no longer respected. The day before diagnosis I was a senior Australian federal public servant. The day after I had become a label: dementia.

Like my friends in DASNI, I was expected to withdraw from the world's stage and be assigned only the smallest walk-on parts. For me it seemed as if from then on I would only ever be allowed to function with my 'carer' in attendance.

But does it have to be that way?

There is life after diagnosis!

Not giving up, nor covering up, although our lives changed forever.

We challenge you with our level of functioning, but are we really that exceptional?

What if we were given rehabilitation and a vital hope of future possibilities?

We reject 'hospice in slow motion'.

We want to come out of the shadows and live positively with dementia!

By writing and giving talks, we challenge the view that people with dementia lack insight, ability or judgement. We are not giving up, nor covering up. Although we retain our ability to present in public using carefully prepared notes, we are open about the diseases that have caused our dementia and drastically changed our lifestyles.

I cannot enjoy busy places because I become fatigued by background noise and motion. Nor can I be left alone in a normal work place, because my judgement is unreliable and my memory extremely unreliable.

You might think that we are somehow misdiagnosed or the disease hasn't hit us, or that our ability to function in giving talks is so exceptional that it is irrelevant to other people with dementia. But what if we were young persons who had suffered head trauma in a motor accident and had analogous diffuse brain damage? And suppose we had parents who paid for the best rehabilitation programs and gave us a vital hope that we could recover rich and productive lives. Our success then would not be so strange.

But all that is given to us is 'hospice in slow motion'. We reject this. We want to come out of the shadows and live positively with dementia!

Let's open the door…

…out of the shadows to a wider world
of possibilities!

No longer in our prison of helpless
victim or hopeless pretender.

No shame in being a person with
dementia – the shame would be in
covering up.

What if we retain neuroplasticity?
What if we could throw off the role of
victim?

We can discover a survivor mission!

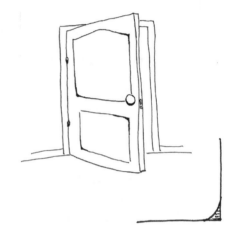

Let's open the door and come out of the shadows to a wider world of possibilities, despite our limitations. No longer enclosed in the prison of helpless victim or hopeless pretender, we can find a new identity, living positively with dementia.

There is no shame in being a person with dementia – the shame would be in covering up. Neither pretending to be normal nor withdrawing into helplessness, we can look to a new future.

What if we retain neuroplasticity? What if we could throw off the role of victim? We can do therapeutic tasks in which failure is unlikely and through which we can start to recover our shattered sense of competence. We can discover ways of giving and caring which restore our sense of value and meaning. We can be recognized and included, by contributing to and participating in the activities of an Alzheimer's association. Thus strengthened, dignified and affirmed, we can face and surmount challenges, with courage and dignity.

Our family is released from a role as denier or carer, and can walk alongside us as we rediscover who we can be. We can discover a survivor mission.

NOTHING ABOUT US, WITHOUT US!

Our survivor mission

We suffer a 'degenerating sense of nobodiness'...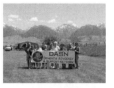

- ▸ ...but aspire to be a great people 'who injected new meaning and dignity into the veins of civilization'

We look forward to a future in which dementia has lost its toxic power:

- ▸ A world focused on relationships
- ▸ with a cure for dementia!

We know what it feels like to have the 'degenerating sense of nobodiness' that oppressed Martin Luther King's fellow black Americans. Yet we have once been normal, like you. Having survived becoming a person with dementia, we know our strength. Our cognition may be fading, but we can draw on powerful resources – our emotions and our spirituality – to relate to you.

We are inspired by Martin Luther King's formulation of his people's survivor mission:

> If you will protest courageously and yet with dignity and Christian love, when the history books are written in future generations, the historians will have to pause and say: there lived a great people – a black people – who injected new meaning and dignity into the veins of civilization.[2]

People with dementia also aspire to be such a people. So what is our vision for the new millennium? We remember when cancer was the dreaded 'C word', and we are inspired by cancer survivors. We look forward to a new future in which the 'D word' of dementia – or that 'A word' of Alzheimer's – has lost its toxic power to create victims.

---

2   This was part of a speech King made during the bus boycott in Montgomery, Alabama on 5 December 1955. It was cited by Gunnar Jahn, chairman of the Nobel Committee on 10 December 1964 (www. nobelprize.org/nobel_prizes/peace/laureates/1964/press.html).

In this new future, people with cognitive difficulties will seek out diagnosis as early as possible, and there will be a cure for all those diseases that cause dementia! In the meantime, as we work towards this goal, they will be prescribed anti-dementia drugs and retain function at the highest possible level for as long as possible. They will remain positive and have support and encouragement.

But ultimately our vision is of a world without dementia!

A dream of future possibilities

My book *Dancing with Dementia* speaks of our dance with you, our care-partners, to adjust to the changing music of dementia.

It's not impossible for us to work with you to realize our dream...of dementia survival with dignity, while we look forward to a cure.

As dementia survivors, by writing books and giving talks, we are companions on this journey.

We want to come out of the shadows and work with you to achieve our dream!

Inspired by the people with dementia that I had met around the world, and the dream I have of a better future, I wrote my second book, *Dancing with Dementia*.[3] It captures our dance, our faltering steps with our care-partners, to adjust to the changing music of dementia. We can shine despite our limitations.

We have a dream of future possibilities. It's harder for us – but not impossible. By writing books and giving talks, and through living positively with dementia, we are companions on this journey towards these future possibilities.

As dementia survivors, we know both the world of 'normals' and that of dementia intimately, and we have weathered an extraordinary transition. We want you to help us realize our dream, where there is dementia survival with dignity, and where we can be one day cured. We want to come out of the shadows and work with you to achieve our dream.

Thank you.

---

3   Christine Bryden (2005) *Dancing with Dementia: My Story of Living Positively with Dementia*. London: Jessica Kingsley Publishers.

12

A decade of change

Christine Bryden

May 2011[1]

It's ten years now since I gave a plenary address to the national conference. It was in Canberra in 2001, and in exactly the same time slot – the first talk on the last day, when many of you are still in recovery from the night before!

So much has changed since then, and since I was first diagnosed. There is now so much more support, inclusion and encouragement. In this talk I will speak about what it was like when I was diagnosed 16 years ago, then describe the changes that have happened in the last decade, and finally look at what we might still need to do.

So what was it like for me at the very beginning of my journey with dementia?

---

1   Plenary presentation to the 11th Alzheimer's Australia National Conference, Brisbane, May 2011, ten years after Christine and Morris Friedell were the first people with dementia to address the Alzheimer's Australia National Conference. Christine also delivered this talk to other State Alzheimer's associations.

Alone with my fear

Diagnosed in 1996 at age 46:

> ▸ single, two young daughters at home.

Life changed overnight, fearful of my future.

Alzheimer's Australia supported only carers.

Stereotype of mindless empty shell:

> ▸ Would that really be me? How soon?

> ▸ What would happen to my girls?

Wrote about my fear in *Who will I be when I die?*

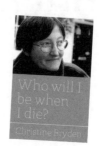

I was only 46 when I was diagnosed in 1995. My life changed overnight and I was very frightened about my future. I had to retire from my job and try to face up to a life of perhaps rapid decline. My neurologist prepared me for the possibility of not being able to write within a year. As a single mother with three daughters aged nine and 14 at home, and a 19-year-old away at university, this was awful.

My first approach to Alzheimer's Australia was a tentative phone call in 1996, when I was asked who I was caring for. When I said it was me, they told me they only had support for carers. I had no one – I was supposed to be the one caring for my daughters.

All I knew was the stereotype of the late stage of dementia, the mindless empty shell of an old person in a nursing home. Would that really be me? How soon? What would happen to my girls? I was left to deal with these fears alone. I became depressed and anxious. But a dear friend encouraged me to write about my feelings, meeting with me regularly to encourage and support me. After a year or so, my first book emerged – with the title capturing my fear of 'Who will I be when I die?' – and was published in 1998.[2] It marked the beginning of remarkable change for me.

---

2   Christine Bryden (2012) *Who will I be when I die?* London: Jessica Kingsley Publishers (first published 1998).

Feeling valued and connected

Less depressed by 1998, chose to be positive.

Approached ACT Alzheimer's for help.

Welcomed by wonderful Michelle McGrath, and met weekly with a few other ladies.

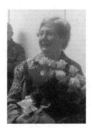

Michelle made me feel like a co-facilitator, she gave me meaning in my life with dementia.

I felt valued and connected.

By early 1998 I had chosen to be as positive as possible, and was trying to overcome my feelings of depression. I decided to approach Alzheimer's Australia again, this time the local ACT office. What a very different response I received! I was welcomed and made to feel valued by the wonderful Michelle McGrath.[3] She gathered together a few other ladies with this diagnosis and we met each week. Sometimes we went out for coffee or shopping; other times we chatted over a cuppa in the ACT office. Michelle made me feel as if I was a co-facilitator and gave me back some meaning in this new life with dementia. I felt valued and connected. I was ready to take my next step in challenging the stereotype of having no hope for my future.

---

3   Former Executive Director of Alzheimer's Australia, ACT.

Steering towards a new future

Married Paul – together we could steer through troubled water of dementia.

Began to speak out in 1999, but:

▸ Was I a freak, not representative of others with dementia?

▸ I was ready to give up.

Meeting in WA about national program of support groups for people with dementia.

I felt part of this new effort.

I went to an introductions agency and met Paul. Married in 1999, together we could steer through the troubled waters of dementia towards a new future. With his support I could do so much more. Together with Michelle, we set up another larger mixed support group, and this received favourable feedback from all participants. A study by Professor Mike Bird showed that attending the group alleviated depression and anxiety.

I began to talk about what it feels like to have dementia, at first to small groups locally, then to the national conference in Western Australia in 1999. But I was not always believed. How could I have dementia if I could speak? Maybe I was a freak, certainly not a credible representative of people with dementia. I really needed Paul alongside me to deal with these challenges to my honesty and credibility. I was ready to give up. It was too hard to keep trying to speak out when some of those who were meant to help did not really believe me.

But there was a very important meeting at that conference. A small group met to talk about a nationally funded program of support groups for people with dementia. Some States had good groups underway, based on the Robyn Yale model,[4] but we wanted to see many more people helped through such groups. Importantly, I felt part of this new effort.

The next year, 2000, was to bring even more change.

---

4   Robyn Yale (1995) *Developing Support Groups for Individuals with Early-Stage Alzheimer's Disease: Planning, Implementation, and Evaluation.* Baltimore, MD: Health Professions Press.

Towards a new future

Glenn Rees brought new vision, building on efforts of the various States.

Consumers of Alzheimer's services, alongside family and professional carers.

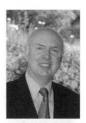

Consumer Working Group – people with dementia – at 2001 conference.

Glenn and Robert Yeoh listened to us. They took action on our recommendations.

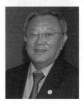

This was the year Glenn Rees became the national executive director. He brought new leadership, building on the achievements of the various States. His was an assertive vision for the future.

Very importantly from the perspective of people with dementia, we became consumers of Alzheimer's services, alongside family carers and professionals. Suddenly, we were being given identity and our views were being listened to.

Glenn asked me to convene a Consumer Working Group of people with dementia at the national conference exactly ten years ago. It was hard at first to get past family carers wondering what I wanted of their loved one. But I managed to gather together a small group from around Australia to meet and discuss what issues were important to us. We reported to the final plenary.

Amazingly, Glenn Rees and the President, Robert Yeoh, came to our final session and listened carefully to what we had to say. Even more amazing to us was the fact that they took action on our recommendations.

One action in particular symbolized what was going to change over the next ten years.

No longer a mindless empty shell!

Logo of Alzheimer's Australia changed to give positive and inclusive image of consumers.

We were all working together for improved services and support.

People with dementia part of narrative.

'Living with dementia' – an ASSERTIVE message.

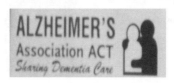 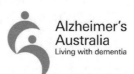

The logo of Alzheimer's Australia was changed to give a positive image of consumers – family and professional carers as well as people with dementia. The strapline says it all; 'Living with dementia'.

No longer were we empty shells, surrounded by the caring arms of others. We were all working together as consumers of Alzheimer's Australia services to improve support for people with dementia and their families.

The new logo is assertive in its symbol and its message. Moving away from the helpless picture of the past, Alzheimer's Australia could advocate for all of those living with dementia. Importantly for us, the voices of people with dementia were at last forming part of the narrative being used to achieve change. Our personal perspectives then became a vital part of one initiative taken by the new-look Alzheimer's Australia.

NOTHING ABOUT US, WITHOUT US!

Dementia – national health priority

Personal stories of those living with dementia appealed to our politicians.

Economic data to back this up.

Parliamentary Friends of Dementia was formed and met with people with dementia, their families and professionals.

Dementia became a national health priority in 2004 – a world first.

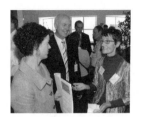

Glenn began to advocate for dementia being recognized as a national health priority. He used the personal stories of people living with dementia and their families to appeal to our politicians. He backed this up with hard economic data from Access Economics[5] about the costs of dementia, and how these would increase in the future.

This assertive approach combining economics and personal testimony was a key factor in attracting the attention of politicians. The Parliamentary Friends of Dementia was formed, giving bipartisan support for our cause. Our politicians began to be able to put a face to our cause by meeting with people living with dementia, their families and professionals.

Dementia became a national health priority in 2004, which was a world first. What did this mean to us as consumers?

Dementia became a national health priority in 2004, which was a world first.

---

5   Beginning in 2003, Alzheimer's Australia commissioned a number of reports from Deloitte Access Economics to research and produce estimates of the current and future impact of dementia in Australia.

Assertive advocacy…

Achieving:

- ▸ Living with Memory Loss program
- ▸ new website
- ▸ consumer advice and participation
- ▸ better services and support.

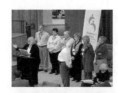
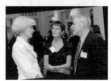

Younger Onset Dementia Summit.

No longer hiding behind negative image of mindless empty shell.

Speaking freely of what matters.

There has been an expansion of services and support for people with dementia and families, including a national program of Living with Memory Loss groups, so that we can be better informed and supported at the start of our journey with dementia. Consumers began to be included in an advisory capacity to Alzheimer's Australia and encouraged through concessional rates and sponsorship to attend and speak at the national conferences. The website was redeveloped, and consumers could access better information, support, services and counselling.

We even had a Younger Onset Dementia Summit in 2009, at which we met the Parliamentary Friends of Dementia, as well as the Governor-General. Our special needs as younger people with dementia were being heard and valued.

The overall message was of being assertive, no longer apologetically hiding behind the negative image set by the stereotype of the mindless empty shell. Assertive advocacy meant that we could now talk freely of what matters to those of us who are living with dementia, and continue to seek improved services and support for all stages in this journey.

But what really matters is what will happen next.

Dementia – disease of society

Fear prevents people seeking early diagnosis and doctors providing treatment for symptoms.

Fear isolates us from friends and social networks.

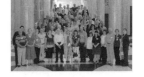

We lack support to deal with our cognitive decline and loss of our place in society.

Cures for the many diseases that result in dementia are still as far away as when I was first diagnosed.

No time to lose to change the stereotype, challenge stigma and fear, and to create a dementia-friendly society.

Dementia is in many ways a disease of society. This disease of society once stopped Alzheimer's Australia from being an effective and assertive advocate on our behalf.

The fear of becoming the stereotype of the mindless empty shell prevents people seeking an early diagnosis. It can also prevent doctors providing treatment, as to do so would mean speaking the word 'dementia', and many doctors are reluctant to burden their patients with this knowledge.

The fear that many people have of dementia, and their discomfort at being with those who have the symptoms, isolates us from our friends and social networks. The tragedy is that in this isolation we are deprived of the support we need to deal with our cognitive decline and loss of our place in society. And cures for the many diseases that result in dementia are still as far away as when I was first diagnosed 16 years ago.

There is no time to lose to change the stereotype, challenge the stigma and fear that results from this, and to begin to create a dementia-friendly society.

My dream: a dementia-friendly society!

Interventions to modify disease progression are as far away as when I was first diagnosed.

Good social support and care will be needed for the hundreds of thousands of people who will be living among us with dementia.

It is up to us, through Alzheimer's Australia, to be assertive in seeking to create a dementia-friendly society in which there is early diagnosis and treatment; and supportive participation in social networks.

We have a strong message and a good story to tell.

My dream is that I will last long enough to see the creation of a dementia-friendly society, in which people will seek and receive early diagnosis, and will receive the best possible treatment for the symptoms of dementia. Isolation will be a thing of the past, as people with dementia are encouraged and supported to participate among family, friends and social networks. By continuing to be assertive in our quest for a dementia-friendly society, we can overcome much of the stigma that isolates and disempowers those with a diagnosis, their families and those around them.

I look back on the last decade and see so much change for the better. If I was diagnosed today, so much of my own and my girls' trauma would be avoided. If I look to the future, for those being diagnosed in ten years' time, I hope and dream for far wider acceptance and inclusion. It is through good social support and care that we will help all of those living with dementia, while we wait for those interventions that might truly modify disease progression, rather than simply help us to cope with a declining level of cognition. These so-called cures are as far away as when I was first diagnosed.

It is up to us, through Alzheimer's Australia, to be assertive in seeking to create a dementia-friendly society that will be needed to support the hundreds of thousands of people who will be living among us with dementia in the next decade. We have a strong message and a good story to tell.

Thank you.

13

Dreading being put in dementia prison

Christine Bryden

November 2012[1]

My talk is based on one I gave to the Aged Care Accreditation Agency, which was then filmed and distributed through the Aged Care Channel. I am so grateful that this was able to be done, as it has meant that many residential care workers throughout Australia have been able to hear my message, and, I hope, think carefully about the standards of care for people with dementia. So if some of my talk sounds familiar, this is why. But I think the message is one that bears repeating. There are not many people with dementia willing or able to speak out, and so when we do, it can give you a unique perspective on what care of people with dementia looks like to us.

I was diagnosed with dementia at the age of only 46, in 1995, yet I'm still here, defying dementia and surviving, trying to speak out for all those who are unwilling or unable to do so. I'm going to try to give you a perspective of residential care from someone who is on a slow but inexorable journey towards being placed in the secure dementia unit – or what I have provocatively called 'dementia prison'.

I would need to go there now without the support I get from my husband, Paul. He is my enabler, encouraging me to keep going and helping me to continue to cope each day. He has helped me become an advocate for people with dementia.

---

1   The Aged Care Standards Agency was responsible for the review of all aged care facilities in Australia against national standards, and their accreditation as registered facilities attracting Government funding. This occasion was their New South Wales Annual Conference (each State has its own conference), bringing together leaders and senior management in the sector. The talk, in Sydney in November 2012, made a deep impression, and Christine was invited by the Agency and many industry groups to deliver it at their conferences across Australia. This version was given in the Gold Coast in July 2013. It was subsequently filmed and, together with later filmed interviews, made into a training DVD distributed to all registered aged care facilities in Australia, where it remains a well-regarded training resource for staff.

Advocacy

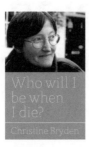

Early signs,
trauma of
diagnosis.

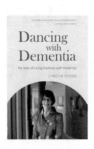

What it feels
like, how you
can help.

I first spoke out a few years after my diagnosis with dementia, when I had managed to overcome depression. I was a divorced mother of three girls aged nine, 13 and 19, and it was a truly awful time for all of us.

Writing my first book, *Who will I be when I die?*,[2] helped me to deal with the trauma of diagnosis. I had been told I would not be expected to last more than around five years before needing full-time residential care, and that I would die a few years later. This was way back in 1995. As you can see, I have defied this prognosis, and intend to keep doing so, with Paul's help, for as long as possible.

I met the lovely Paul in 1998 – but that is a story for another day! Together we spent a few years meeting others living with dementia, and visiting day care and residential care homes. I drew on these national and international experiences to write my second book, *Dancing with Dementia*.[3] It talks of what it feels like for me and for so many of my friends, and what you can do to help us.

Let's now look briefly at the reason for me being here today to give you an insider's perspective.

---

2   Christine Bryden (2012) *Who will I be when I die?* London: Jessica Kingsley Publishers (first published 1998).
3   Christine Bryden (2005) *Dancing with Dementia: My Story of Living Positively with Dementia.* London: Jessica Kingsley Publishers.

My 'credentials'

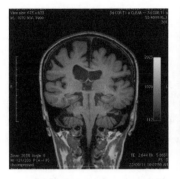
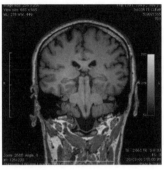

My brain scan...and   ...an age-matched
                             'normal' brain

These high-resolution MRI brain scans, taken in September 2011, are my 'credentials'. My scan on the left is compared with an age-matched normal brain on the right. It's clear that I have significant brain damage, particularly to the frontal and temporal lobes.

My functioning on the testing is also impaired considerably, particularly when compared with the speedy multi-tasking person I once was long ago. It has also declined slowly over the years since diagnosis. The neurologist is extremely puzzled as to why I still function, let alone still speak, given this brain damage. But I will do my best to keep speaking out, on this long journey from diagnosis to death.

One issue in particular
frightens me and ignites
my passion, and that is
the standard of residential
care for dementia.

Behind locked doors

People sit without dignity.

Staff speak loudly to each other.

Occupational therapist with cheery determination for meaningless activities.

TV and radio compete with staff chatter and clatter.

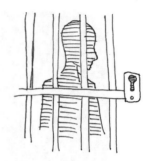

Soon I'm exhausted, blankly staring into space like everyone else!

I have visited quite a few nursing homes now over the years, here and overseas.

Entering the foyer and main areas, at first the impression is bright and airy, cheerful and homely. This delight changes to despair as I enter the secure area. Clearly this is hidden away and not showcased by the nursing home.

I am terrified by what I see. People sit without dignity in chairs at tables, or in lounges. Staff speak loudly to each other, with scant regard for this area being the residents' living room.

The occupational therapist comes in once or twice a week, larger than life in her cheery determination to make residents do activities that seem meaningless.

TV and radio compete with staff chatter.

After an hour or so of visiting, I feel exhausted, needing to sit like the others in the room, blankly staring into space. Then Paul leads me away for some brain 'time out' in the quiet of our home.

How can I tell you?

We communicate our needs by our challenging behaviours.

Am I just an object to be physically cared for by the overworked staff?

It is behind the locked doors that we can judge the standard of palliative care for people with dementia.

Lost in a state of unknowing.

Volunteers are very rare, and even our families seem to have deserted us. The staff are often casuals, or agency, so unfamiliar faces surround us. Few staff really want to work with or deal with our challenging behaviours. And yet these behaviours are all we are left with to communicate our needs. How else can we say we are in pain, we don't like the food, we are hungry or tired, or overwhelmed by noise?

For me, how the dementia unit operates is the benchmark of care.

Men and women are accommodated together, despite behaviours that might be very distressing, such as inappropriate sexual contact and invasion of our privacy. Do I really want some strange man in my living room, or even in my bedroom? Do I really want to be woken up for an early shower, when all my life I have had a warm shower just before bed? Do I really want to feel as if I am no longer human, but simply an object to be physically cared for by the harassed and overworked staff?

The environment is noisy and disabling, making me feel exhausted and confused. Our brain damage can make us feel lost in a state of unknowing – what has happened, what might happen, where am I, why am I here?

For me, how the dementia unit operates is the benchmark of care. Rather than the impressions of the main areas, it is behind the closed doors that we can see palliative care in action.

Our humanity

Like you, we are human beings with emotional and spiritual needs.

We are more than mouths to be fed, bodies to wash and clothe, beds to make.

Help us find meaning, and affirm our humanity as death approaches.

▸ Physical

▸ Emotional

▸ Spiritual

▸ **Palliative care**

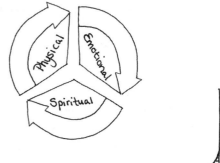

Yes, care of people with dementia is palliative care, although often for longer than is normally the case. So our care needs to affirm our humanity as we approach the end of life, when it is important to reflect, find a sense of meaning and nourish our spirit.

We are human beings just like you, with physical, emotional and spiritual needs. Look around your secure area. Are these being met in equal amounts? Put yourself in our shoes and see what is the same – a need to belong, to have respect and dignity, affection and social interaction, companionship and valued and meaningful activity. Are we regarded as emotional and spiritual beings? Are we thought to have the same needs as you? What about our privacy, time apart with partners for a caress or cuddle?

What actually does happen? The staff of each shift hurriedly try to struggle through an impossible workload of physical care set to a strict schedule. We are mouths to be fed, bodies to wash and clothe, beds to make – little more.

In so doing, our emotional and spiritual needs remain unmet.

So I pose the question to you all: How can this be changed?

Experiential model

Biomedical model – I'm a fatal, tragic and costly pathology.

Experiential model – my experience of dementia is a shift in perception of, and interaction with, the world.

'It's the way you talk to us, not what you say, that we will remember. We know the feelings, but we do not know the plot.'

Is dementia a gift? Stripping away outer masks, are we free in the spirit, to live in the 'now' and to treasure this?

We are people, not disease burdens.

We need to move away from the biomedical model which sees me as my dementia – a fatal pathology which is tragic and costly – towards an experiential model in which my experience of dementia is regarded as a shift in my perception of the world and the way I interact with it. So often we are far more sensitive than you to our surroundings – far better at reading emotions. It is the way you talk to us, not what you say, that we will remember. We know the feelings, but we don't know the plot.

Overcome your fear of dementia and try to change your perception. Can dementia be a gift? What is it like to strip away the outer work of cognition and the emotional masks within, to be free in the spirit, to live in the now and to treasure this?

I challenge you all to help us to find meaning in our lives and to connect with us as people first and foremost, not as a disease burden. There are so many theories and approaches to care for people with dementia, but will I really experience these, or are they just words to cover up the fact that there is not enough time or money to practise them?

Person-centred?

We're sensitive to how a place 'feels' – maybe we can audit your facility?

Are staff kind and appreciative, knowing residents well?

How will our families feel when we move in there?

Does the environment overwhelm or enable us?

So often I hear the words 'person-centred care', but I can't *feel* it happening. Don't forget that people with dementia are very sensitive to how a place *feels*, even in the earlier stages of these diseases that disable us and kill us over time.

Maybe support groups for people with a diagnosis and their families can come and visit your facility? We could 'audit' it for how it feels. Each one of us will need to come into your care sooner or later, or help someone else move into your care, however much we might want to ignore this fact.

We will be looking for autonomy, feeling valued, in relationship with others and our individuality supported. We will be looking to see if all of our needs can be met, not just our immediate physical needs.

Are men and women separated, or all in together, despite our differing behaviours and needs?

We will feel whether the environment overwhelms us with its competing stimuli, or enables us through its quietness and peace, its homely feel.

Do the staff feel kind and appreciative of each resident? Is behaviour watched carefully for its meaning? How will our families feel when we go in there? Will we have ready access to the outside?

Do staff know much about each resident? Is it easy for the next shift to get key information that helps them relate to us as an individual?

'Malignant'?

We are ignored as staff talk among themselves.

We are treated worse than children.

Pace of life outstrips our ability to follow and respond.

We are labelled by dementia.

We sit around waiting: for what, for whom?

Are we disempowered, infantilized, outpaced, labelled, objectified, even ignored?

Are we just a bother to your endless round of time-critical tasks?

Next time, in the secure area, close your eyes and enter into our world. What do you hear? Does it sound and feel like home? Would you want to live here 24 hours a day for the next few years?

Are there signs of Tom Kitwood's malignant social psychology around you? Are we being disempowered, infantilized, outpaced, labelled, objectified, even ignored? Kitwood came up with 17 of these interactions that erode our personhood.[4] These are only some of them, the ones I see and feel most often when I visit the secure area.

Tasks are hurriedly performed and we are not encouraged to do much at all except sit around waiting – for what, for whom?

We are ignored as staff talk among themselves, over us and around us, excluding us. We are treated worse than children, patronized rather than respected or delighted in. The pace of life during our daily routine outstrips our ability to follow and respond.

We sense we are labelled by our disease, no longer remembered for who we once were – and still are! Everything we do or say is because of our dementia, not an expression of how we feel. We are just a bother to the endless round of time-critical tasks.

How can I hope for better, given the constraints of time and money?

---

4   Tom Kitwood was a pioneer who tried to understand what care is like from the standpoint of the person with dementia. Published in 1997 by Open University Press, his book *Dementia Reconsidered: The Person Comes First* speaks of harmful care in terms of malignant social psychology.

Enabling environment

Colours and tones muted and harmonious.

No visual clutter in main area: it needs to be restful!

Floors same colour and texture.

Lighting adequate but not harsh.

Access to outside, with comfy chairs.

Don't over-stimulate!

I don't want to be over-stimulated, and I've never yet met a person with dementia who does, especially by noise and motion. In such a disabling environment, much of my time will be spent gazing blankly into space as my brain shuts down and I feel weariness rise within me. Maybe that's when you will want to stimulate me, as I seem to be apathetic?

Colours need to be muted and the tones harmonious. No fussy couches or curtains, or garishly modern pieces. Visual clutter is very disturbing, so minimize the bits and pieces around in our living room. Of course we will want our memorabilia around us in our bedroom, but the main area needs to be restful, as it has enough things and people in it already!

Floors need to be the same colour and texture, so as not to disturb our field of vision when we are trying to walk. Lighting should be adequate but not harsh during the day and dimmed a little in the evening to help us sense a restful time is approaching. Access to outside should be available, with comfy chairs, a bird feeder perhaps, and flowers and herbs to look at.

But far more important are the people who care for us!

'Being alongside'

Familiar faces around me.

Care plan developed in my team approach with my family and volunteers as part of a circle of care.

Sit with me, having eye contact, touching my hand and listening.

Good CARE of people with dementia is like chaplaincy.

Like chaplaincy, good care for people with dementia is about 'being alongside' a person. It's about sitting with me, having eye contact, touching my hand and listening. I want to have familiar faces around me, and sense a true connection with them. Staff need to want to be there – to have a calling to this special care. Agency staff cannot usually offer us this.

Maybe you could look at involving volunteers, who can bring valuable life experience to the task. Simple training can help them have the confidence they will need. Maybe my care plan can be developed and implemented in cooperation with my family, who feel relaxed and welcomed as they visit my new home?

Sometimes we may need smaller secure units to suit the types of people being cared for. Are the people I am sharing my home with those I would normally have met in my day-to-day life? Are they very differently affected by their dementia? Are they violent, aggressive, disturbing? Would you want to live with them?

The key to my care will be effective communication with me, listening and reflecting, even though my ways of responding might be impaired.

Communication

Non-verbal facial expression, body language.

What's causing my behaviour? Look for clues before saying I'm difficult, especially when 'things need to be done and done quickly'.

Everything we do and utter is communication and is often unheard.

Violence is the voice of the unheard.

Much of our communication is the same as yours, such as facial expression and body language. These non-verbal clues can tell an observant person a great deal.

What is causing my non-verbal communication – what you might call challenging behaviour? Am I in discomfort or suffering in any way? I don't want to be left in pain, or given food that I dislike or am not given enough time to chew, just because I can't tell you this clearly.

Look for clues before saying I am difficult, especially when 'things need to be done and done quickly'. There is so little time and so much to do. But physical care is often intimate, so don't embarrass me or rush me. Respect me and maybe try candles and calm music as if I am at the beauty therapist. Remember to slow down and talk me quietly through it. Knock, sit, listen, slow down and connect. Could the physical care tasks be done in small bits through the day, each time being an opportunity for meaningful interaction?

Everything we do and utter is a way of communicating, which so often goes unheard. People with dementia, whose communication is impaired, can really relate to Martin Luther King's words that 'Violence is the voice of the unheard.'[5]

---

5   Christine paraphrased the original quote by Martin Luther King, 'A riot is the language of the unheard'. This was part of a speech King made to Grosse Point High School on 14 March 1986, called 'The other America' (www.gphistorical.org).

Meaningful interaction

Dementia is a disease of communication, creating a barrier between us.

Draw on my life history to find appropriate activities, based on your insight and respect.

PAUSE...for me to work out what you're saying.

I need TIME to make pictures in my head (like thought balloons) into words or gestures.

Having dementia significantly impairs my ability to communicate. Perhaps we can say dementia is a disease of communication, creating an unseen barrier between your world and mine, which your intuition can breach. Take time to listen, use pauses to give me time to process what you are saying, and how to make the pictures in my head into gestures, facial expression or words for you to understand. It may feel very odd at first, to do this, but it would enable me to connect with you.

Don't be afraid to experiment to find things for me to do that make your life easier – that settle me down, or make my life more meaningful as I approach my last days. I have a rich life history and wisdom to share which can make our interaction one of insight and respect. It can be drawn on in developing meaningful and engaging activities. Please don't simply entertain me with movies, bingo, sing-alongs.

> Ask yourself: What would
> you like to do if you
> were in my place?

What would I have done in the past? Can this be in my care plan? Can my family help? They too will then gain a sense of being valued and fulfilled. Focus on what I can still do, rather than on what I can't do. How can I help others? How can I help you? In this way I will feel valued in my new home.

Nurture spirit

IQ and EQ are no measure of my relationship with the divine.[6]

The meaning of my life is to be in relationship with Jesus…increasingly so as masks of cognition and emotion fade.

Encourage normal spiritual practices as I near end of life.

**I am who I am – I am not a lost soul,
nor am I no longer there.**

I am created in the image of God.

I am not my dementia – I am who I am, created in the image of God. I am not a lost soul, nor am I no longer there. The scrambling of my cognitive and emotional abilities has not diminished my spirit, nor my relationship with the divine.

For me, the meaning of my life is to be in relationship with Jesus, and this may well become even stronger as the masks of cognition and emotion fall away further to reveal my inner spirit. So please don't exclude me from my normal spiritual practices. So often the religious services are held in the main nursing home. Because of a lack of staff, people from the secure area rarely, if ever, attend. And the volunteers offering these services are not invited or trained to come in to minister to us.

Yet it is all the more critical for us to receive nurture to our spirits, very importantly with respect for our past beliefs and practices. Some of us may never have had a formal religious belief, but felt a sense of the divine in music, nature or art. Whatever truly gave us a sense of purpose and meaning in life needs to be drawn on to minister to us.

Care of people with dementia is palliative care, as I said before. It is now, as we approach the end of our life, that we need to be helped to find meaning.

---

6   Intelligence quotient (IQ) is a number representing a person's reasoning ability, which is calculated using problem-solving tests. The number relates to the statistical norm or average for the person's age, which is taken as 100. Emotional quotient (EQ) is a number representing a person's emotional intelligence, often determined by their score in a standardized test.

My dream…

My secure area is welcoming and inviting.

My own unique life story guides my circle of care.

Look at BENEFITS as well as risks.

Courtyard style security…allowing access to outside.

Walking and pottering, not wandering!

My dream is that my secure area – my new home – will be a showcase of true person-centred care, ministering to my physical, emotional and spiritual needs. It will be as welcoming and inviting as the 'normal' residential areas. I will have my own unique life story on my door – just a few key points in addition to a folder kept in the office – so that staff and volunteers caring for me can relate to me in a more meaningful way.

There is information on dementia-enabling environments, and often just simple changes can achieve them. When I am inside, I would like the choice of spaces that feel like a lounge or a dining room, and to be able to move away from noise such as TV or radio when I need quiet time to rest. I won't feel vulnerable to aggression or sexual advances from strange men, and I will be surrounded by women. I want to be able to have a choice to sit outside, maybe sipping a decent coffee, under shelter in a comfy chair, looking perhaps at a bird feeder, flowers and herbs. Nature has such a calming effect on me!

Rooms set around a secure courtyard would be ideal, giving me freedom to walk. I don't want to be locked into a chair just because I have osteoporosis. Let's look at the benefits, not just the risks. I want to feel free to go for a short walk. Let's change the language and call this walking, as that is what everyone else does. It's only when I potter around in my new home that it will be called wandering!

No answers, just dreams

There are costs, time and staffing constraints.

Maybe space out physical tasks, include family and volunteers?

Relationships, not money.

Failure to attend to the whole person can cost more $$$$$$$$.

Mature, confident…in relationship with you.

Why not?

I want to be dressed nicely and look like a mature and confident woman. But I don't want to be rushed first thing in the morning. Surely I can stay in my PJs for a while?

I want to have colourful food – not necessarily tasty or aromatic – that is easy to chew. I want time to eat, as chewing and swallowing are no longer easy or automatic. And what about a glass of wine with my evening meal? Why should I suddenly become a teetotaller in my last days, without the glass of wine to calm me down at the end of the day, when you refer to me as showing 'sun-downing'?

I want to do meaningful activities, such as going on outings, making useful things and being included in the main nursing home activities, especially the Sunday services. I don't want to be excluded because of lack of staff. Let's look at a circle of care involving family and volunteers.

I don't have the answers as to how all my dreams can be fulfilled, for I realize that there are costs, time and staffing constraints. But failure to attend to each one of us as a whole human being with emotional and spiritual needs – as well as simply physical needs – can be more costly in the long term. It's all about relationships – not about money.

While I dream of a better future, I'll try to change your perception of care of people with dementia. It's really very simple to do.

Put yourself in our shoes

You've moved to new home for the limited time you've left on earth.

Is this where you want to be?

What would you ask, if you could still speak?

Talk about dementia care in first person: it's your last move ever!

Will you feel welcome in your new home?

Will you want to move in?

What would YOU want?

Just start talking about care for people with dementia in the first person. Put yourself in our shoes. Unable to communicate clearly what you want, it's like being in a foreign country. You've entered into a new world that is going to be your home for the limited time that you have left on this earth. Is this where you want to be? If you could speak clearly, what would you say? What would you ask of your family and friends if you could still make yourself understood?

There are so many approaches to care of people with dementia, which all speak of putting the person first before his or her disease. But do they look at all aspects of our humanity? Even if they are practised throughout the nursing home, do they reach beyond those locked doors, of what I have provocatively called 'dementia prison'?

All I ask today is for you to try to become – for even a short moment – the person with dementia who is living within these walls. Care of people with dementia is a huge challenge, but one which I hope will be met before I need to join my friends in the secure area.

Eventually, Paul and I will choose a nursing home, based on what I see and feel around me as I enter the dementia ward, not the main foyer. Will I feel welcome in my new home? Will I want to move in? Would you want to join me there? Think about this for a while, as if it were also your choice to make. It's over to you now to find ways to make some of my dreams possible.

Thank you.

14

Living life to the full

Christine Bryden

October 2013[1]

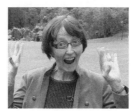

I am extremely honoured today to be giving this address on the occasion of the launch of Uniting AgeWell.

I'm Christine Bryden, a person living with dementia. Yes, I know that in this picture it looks as if this diagnosis is well deserved, but it does express my joy of living each day to the full! I take great comfort and strength from Jesus' words: 'I have come that they may have life and have it to the full.' And I am sure that He meant I could have lots of fun along the way!

Today I plan to give a little bit of background about me, and then talk about some issues. I will reflect on current models of care, as well as look at ways I'd like to see these improved.

I welcome the exciting new approach of Uniting AgeWell. I believe it will support us with dignity, honour and respect – maybe with fun and zest for life as well – when we approach our later years. It will also support us on our journey of decline and disability with a range of terminal illnesses, including dementia. Let's look at when I began to reflect on all of these things from an insider's point of view.

---

1   The Uniting Church agency Uniting Aged Care invited Christine to launch their rebranding to 'Uniting AgeWell' in Melbourne, October 2013.

Biomedical approach

Told: five years till you become demented, about another three years in care till you die.

Scans – my potent symbol of life transformed by biomedical approach.

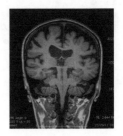

BUT:

‣ Over 100 diseases cause dementia.

‣ Each person has a unique life history, education, personality.

It's possible to live a new life in the slow lane of dementia!

I was diagnosed with Alzheimer's at the age of 46, and three years later this was revised to fronto-temporal dementia. I was told the standard biomedical prognosis: 'You have about five years till you become demented, and then around three years in care till you die.' My scan is a potent symbol of a life transformed by this biomedical approach. The dismal prognosis was a truly awful thing to hear at the age of 46! And it was a huge shock and a traumatic time for me and my young daughters.

But such a clinical approach assumes that our brains, our life histories and our individual life experiences are all the same. It assumes that the damage to our brains will occur at the same rate, no matter which disease we have, despite there being more than a hundred different diseases, each affecting the brain in different ways and yet each causing the symptoms of dementia.

I sought a second opinion, as I was convinced I was far too young to have dementia. This neurologist saw me as a unique individual, and although he confirmed the diagnosis, he gave me hope. He said he could not predict the future, but that I should immediately begin taking anti-dementia medication, and do the best I could, for as long as I could.

When I meet people who are just going through that awful time of diagnosis, I try to give them hope by saying it is possible to live a new life in the slow lane of dementia. As part of this new life, I think it is very important to find purposeful activity.

I'm still here!

Finding purpose in advocacy (talks, books, travels).

Paul enables me to keep speaking out, giving an insider's view.

'Christine effect' in Japan.

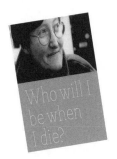 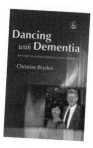

For me, this has been my advocacy for people with dementia, here in Australia and around the world. I often say, 'I'm still here!' as people do not expect me to still be defying those medical expectations. My first book, *Who will I be when I die?*,[2] published in 1998, launched me somewhat reluctantly on this path of speaking out for all those who do not want to (public speaking is one of people's greatest fears!). I also know that I am speaking out for those who are no longer able to do so. In my talks I try to describe what it feels like to have dementia and what you can do to help. It's an insider's perspective, and one that makes me unusual as a speaker, but makes me a credible advocate for people with dementia here and elsewhere.

Luckily for me, by the time I needed to travel as an advocate for people with dementia, I had Paul by my side to support me. He is my enabler, helping me cope as best I can, despite my steady decline. I met him in 1998, and talk about this love story in my second book *Dancing with Dementia*,[3] published in 2005. I describe how we met through an introductions agency (of course, I didn't tell them my diagnosis; otherwise I would never have been introduced to the lovely Paul).

---

2   Christine Bryden (2012) *Who will I be when I die?* London: Jessica Kingsley Publishers (first published 1998).

3   Christine Bryden (2005) *Dancing with Dementia: My Story of Living Positively with Dementia*. London: Jessica Kingsley Publishers.

It has been a truly amazing journey of advocacy, taking us around the world several times, and many times to Japan, where the 'Christine effect' has apparently given people with dementia recognition and respect. My books have now been translated into several languages, and I regularly receive emails from around the world from people who have been diagnosed or who have a person close to them who has dementia. It has been wonderful to hear how the books have helped people living with dementia and their families understand what it feels like to have dementia and what can be done to help.

Decline and despair

Multiple losses:

- abilities
- role in society
- meaningful activity

which all lead to a loss of identity.

Death stares you in the face.

Life feels so short and devoid of purpose.

Pastoral care to carry our broken emotions and heal our spirit.

Who am I when I no longer 'do' things?

Why am I here? What's it all been about?

But don't let me give the breezy impression that it was easy to become positive and purposeful after my diagnosis! It took nearly three years of despair, depression and some really bleak times, during which I was trying to write my first book. I was trying to make sense of what was happening to me and my three young daughters, who were only aged 19, 14 and nine. I drew on fantastic support from my church family, and searched the depths of my Christian faith to find hope and a sense of meaning in this dark turmoil.

For so many people, a diagnosis of a terminal illness like mine, or when they are approaching their later years and they go to more funerals than weddings, is really a dismal time. You face multiple losses – of abilities, of a role in society, of meaningful activity at work and at home – which all lead to a loss of identity. Who am I when I no longer can 'do' things?

We feel disempowered, and experience despair, leading to depression. Life becomes an absence of hope and an absence of meaning in life. Death stares you in the face, and life feels so short and devoid of purpose. Why am I here? What's it all been about?

We need your help to cope with mounting devastation in our lives. We need pastoral care that gently carries our broken emotions and heals our spirits. But what is offered to us in this time of decline and despair? What surrounds us in society as we struggle to carry on coping in our own homes?

Stigma disables us

Negativity in society towards old age and dementia.

Double whammy of stigma.

Stigma around us and within us, so we feel shame, exclusion and discrimination.

Language has great power to tear down or to lift up – to demean us or to encourage us.

We are the experts in our own lived experience of ageing and of disease – always affirm us and encourage us.

It's stigma created through negative language and feelings about us. The negative views in society of old age result in us feeling shame, exclusion and discrimination. Then, if we also have dementia, we have the stigma of this illness to cope with as well, which results in the classic double whammy.

Stigma is pervasive in society, and in turn creates a stigma within us, as we feel worthless and of little value. We withdraw from trying to continue to function. Not only are we isolated by our disability or lack of mobility, but we are also isolated by stigma. We may well receive home visits, meals on wheels or a shower nurse, but all these interactions can be affected by the negative power of language.

Language has great power to tear down or to lift up – to demean us or to encourage us. Don't patronize us by coming out with such phrases as 'That always happens to me' or 'I often feel that way'. How could that be true unless you too were elderly or had a disease such as dementia? Don't forget we are the experts in our own lived experience of ageing and of disease. Always affirm us and encourage us.

So often the struggle of coping alone at home – which is something most of us face – ends in a crisis such as a fall or illness. And then we transition – a polite way of saying a huge and traumatic change in our lives – to a greater level of care, usually in the residential care sector.

The old way…

…can smother us, not enable us.

It's all about physical care as objects to be got up, showered, dressed and parked at tables.

We have become invisible, depersonalized and dehumanized.

Outpacing us is all too easy to do, as we are so very slow.

We are treated worse than children, as, unlike them, we are not delighted in!

The old way of giving us this support can smother us, not enable us. It's all about our physical care – as objects to be got up, showered, dressed and sat around tables. Somehow we have become invisible, depersonalized and dehumanized. Tom Kitwood[4] observed this and described 17 signs of what he called 'malignant social psychology' in our care environment, which erodes our personhood. Let's look at just two of the 17 signs of this that he came up with – ones that are readily seen in residential care.

---

4   Tom Kitwood was a pioneer who tried to understand what care is like from the standpoint of the person with dementia. Published in 1997 by Open University Press, his book *Dementia Reconsidered: The Person Comes First* speaks of harmful care in terms of malignant social psychology.

Tom Kitwood's malignant social psychology

- Accusation
- Banishment
- Disempowerment
- Disparagement
- Disruption
- Ignoring
- Imposition
- Infantilization
- Intimidation

- Invalidation
- Labelling
- Mockery
- Objectification
- Outpacing
- Stigmatization
- Treachery
- Withholding

Outpacing us is all too easy to do as we are so slow. It is so much quicker to do things for us, rather than with us. But then we stop doing things and give up. Another sign is **infantilizing**. Yet I think we are treated worse than children, as children are delighted in; we are not.

A friend of mine – let's call her Barb – went into residential care earlier this year. She is furious at being called 'dearie'. She says: 'My name is Barb, not Barbara, and certainly not lovey, not dearie!' Her first few months were spent in tears as she felt she had lost her former identity, as a lady with intellect, humour and great strength of character. Now she must fight each day to retain her dignity.

Let's now look at ways to categorize residential care, and I will draw on the models used by Dr Cameron Camp.[5]

---

5   American Montessori expert Dr Cameron Camp promoted Alzheimer's Australia's Quality Dementia Care resource *Relate, Motivate, Appreciate: Restoring Meaningful Engagement with a Person with Dementia in Care* with a lecture tour in all capital cities across Australia during July through until September 2013.

Hotel model

Everything is done for you: we lose our ability to do things ourselves.

Maria Montessori said: 'Everything you do for me, you take away from me.'

Use it or lose it.

Neuroplasticity – we can keep rewiring even as our brain is unwiring.

Need enablers beside us, as our cheerleaders, encouragers and helpers.

The first can be seen as a hotel, where everything is done for us. We do not normally live in a hotel, although it's great for a short break. The thought of living in a hotel sounds grand, but it is extremely disabling.

Maria Montessori said: 'Everything you do for me, you take away from me.' I have often referred to this loss of function as 'use it or lose it'. So often we hear that people go rapidly downhill after they have entered into residential care.

I believe that if we keep trying to do things, even as our brain is unwiring, we can rewire new bits to take over functions that are being lost. This neuroplasticity can only be achieved if we keep trying to do things, with enablers beside us, as our cheerleaders, as our encouragers, and as helpers, should we need a bit of prompting along the way.

I think the reason I can keep talking, writing and reading – even though my brain is very damaged – is that I have kept on trying very hard to do these functions, with Paul alongside to cheer me on. He does not write or talk for me. If I no longer had access or encouragement to keep trying, I am sure I would rapidly lose these abilities.

Now for another disabling model.

Prison model

No choice but to shower and get dressed, eat and sit at times not of your own choosing.

Our lives regimented 'for the term of our natural lives'.

What meaning is left in life if there is no choice or no freedom?

Prison model results in apathy, boredom and hopelessness.

This is the prison, where you are given no choice but to shower and get dressed, eat and sit at times not of your own choosing. Behind locked doors, like those you see leading to the dementia ward, we sit with our lives regimented 'for the term of our natural lives'.

Paul is a prison chaplain, and he sees the reality of this model in his work – prisoners looking despondent, sitting with nothing to do and yet all the time to do it. What meaning is left in life if there is no choice or no freedom? Even small choices such as whether to have coffee or tea will make us feel in control of our lives. What results from the prison model is apathy, boredom and hopelessness.

Have you seen apathy in the faces of those in residential care? This withdrawal from life is extremely disabling and leads to rapid decline.

Now for the third model, which is equally disabling.

Hospital model

Visually, a nurses' station and long corridor with very similar doors all along.

Functionally, given medications and vital signs are checked.

Have you been in hospital for a few days or more? Did you feel weak when you got home?

What if you had to stay in hospital for the rest of your life?

This is the hospital model, which is so common in the residential care sector. It is based on the biomedical approach to our treatment.

Visually, there is a nurses' station and a long corridor with very similar doors all along. Functionally, we are given medications, and our vital signs are checked daily.

Have you been in hospital for a few days or more? Did you feel weak when you got home? What if you had to stay in the hospital for the rest of your life?

These three models of care – hotel, prison and hospital – are each disabling. Even in our own home, the stigma that surrounds us in society also disables us.

So how can we move towards enabling people in their later years and those with terminal illnesses?

There is a new way…'home'

'The best place to be if I can't be at home.'

Give us choice. Focus on wellness. Enable us to have hope.

Focus on what I can do, reaffirming my wellness.

Empower us on our journey towards death, finding ways to overcome deficits.

Create 'moments of wellbeing'.

We need your empowering care to find abundant life, enjoying each day as it comes.

We can live life to the full, finding meaning and purpose as well as hope.

There is a new way of caring for us, enabling us to age well and to face death well. I call this the 'home model'. My mother described her care home as 'the best place to be if I can't be at home'.

- Give us choice.
- Focus on wellness.
- Enable us to have hope.

Focus on what I can do, reaffirming my wellness, not my disease or my ageing. Empower us on our journey towards death, finding ways to overcome any of our deficits. For example, I need to be provided with 'cognitive ramps'. Don't ask me to remember an event. Instead, describe your own memories, so that you have created a word picture for me to walk into and gather up a few fragments of my own recollection to share this memory with you.

Create moments of wellbeing throughout my day; it is not important that I remember the log of activities, but rather enjoy each moment as it goes by.

We need your empowering care to find abundant life, enjoying each day as it comes. We can live life to the full, finding meaning and purpose, as well as hope.

Create an enabling environment

Social engagement – we are social beings, finding meaning in relationship with others.

Embedded in a complex network of relationships, with familiar strangers in our neighbourhood, other residents and staff.

We play a vital social role in this community and recapture our identity.

You 'listen with your eyes', watching our non-verbal communication.

An important part of this empowering care is creating an enabling environment, which includes social engagement. Humans are social beings, finding meaning in relationship with others. We function best in a network of relationships, whether that is with familiar strangers in our neighbourhood, other residents or staff. Within this community we play a social role and recapture our identity.

Importantly, our behaviour will be recognized as non-verbal communication. You will be listening with your eyes, watching for any sign that the environment is overwhelming us or disempowering us. Our behaviour should never be seen as challenging, but responsive to the environment around us. Ask yourself 'Why is this happening?' Are we in discomfort or pain? Are we hungry? Can we chew and swallow at the speed you expect us to? Are we bored or overwhelmed by noise or visual stimuli?

The enabling environment will be a community of clients, family and staff with the mutual goal of living life with hope and finding meaning in life.

Let's examine how we can regard each person as more than just a physical object.

Created in the image of God

I am created in the image of God, with body, mind and spirit.

As my physical and cognitive abilities decrease, so there can be more of my spirit self revealed to you.

I am removing masks that once defined me; deep within, my spirit remains intact.

Despite my multiple losses, you can relate to me spirit to spirit, and, in so doing, restore my sense of self.

Lord, make me an instrument of your peace.

Where there is hatred, let me sow love;

where there is injury, pardon;

where there is doubt, faith;

where there is despair, hope;

where there is darkness, light;

and where there is sadness, joy.

I am created in the image of God, and have a body, mind and spirit. As my physical abilities decrease, so my mind and my spirit can increase. As I lose my cognitive self, so there can be more of my spirit self revealed to you.

As I age, as I decline with dementia, my spirit can flourish as an important source of identity. So, throughout my journey of life, and especially through the ravages of dementia, I am removing masks that once defined me. First I remove the mask of my status in terms of my job and other roles in society. Then I must remove my emotional mask, as that becomes more unpredictable in my journey towards death. Deep within, my spirit remains intact, despite the toll that has been taken in this journey of ageing or disease.

Despite my multiple losses, you can relate to me spirit to spirit and, in so doing, restore my sense of self. Never forget that I am a full human being – body, mind and spirit – just like you. In the words of St Francis of Assisi, may you be instruments of God's peace, sowing the seeds of love, pardon, faith, hope, light and joy. We need holistic and empowering care, with you alongside us as our enablers in restoring our wholeness.

A new way of thinking: Uniting AgeWell

Underpins restorative wellness model like the one I described as 'home'

Environment of choice, empowerment and wellness

Enhances life experience

Enables choice and independence

Emphasizes our abilities within the community

Expresses Church's response to the vulnerable and disadvantaged

Values of respect, partnership, wisdom, stewardship and fairness shape this life-enhancing approach to ageing and disease.

The new way of thinking to be offered through Uniting AgeWell underpins a restorative wellness model. This model is like the one I described as 'home', as it offers an environment of choice, empowerment and wellness. It is amazing that your new approach aligns so closely with what I have been thinking and talking about for some time. It:

- enhances life experience
- enables choice and independence
- emphasizes our abilities within the community
- expresses the Church's response to the vulnerable and disadvantaged, by attending to our spiritual and pastoral needs.

Values of respect, partnership, wisdom, stewardship and fairness shape this life-enhancing approach to ageing and disease. I feel honoured today to be able to be at this launch of a revolutionary new way of thinking – one that will transform the lives of so many who are seeking true meaning and purpose as they near the end of their lives. What a blessing you will be to so many people and their families.

Thank you.

15

Mind your language – getting it right!

Christine Bryden

November 2014[1]

I'm going to talk to you this afternoon about what it feels like as a consumer – or to be a patient of yours – when you speak to us or about us.

Over the many years since my diagnosis with dementia, some of my experiences with clinicians have been truly shocking, and often it is their language that has made the most impact. And, equally, my interactions with sympathetic clinicians, who are careful about how they speak to me and what words they use, have made the most positive impression.

We hear your language acutely – and also we read your body language. So it's not just a matter of studying what words to say but how to say them that will make your clinical relationship with us work or not. It's not always what you say, but how you say it. But today I will cover the words that you use, and I hope by looking at this issue of language through the lens of someone with dementia, it will help you to consider how best to interact with us.

---

1 Christine is one of two Consumer Members of the Steering Committee of the Queensland Statewide Dementia Clinical Network, which brings together 200 or more specialists and clinicians in the public and private medical systems for twice-yearly face-to-face forums. This talk was presented in Brisbane in November 2014 and promotes the Dementia Language Guidelines recently released by Alzheimer's Australia.

Talk2Me!

Suddenly I'm invisible!

Please talk to me – I am not deaf, nor a mindless empty shell.

Make eye contact, use simple clear language.

Make sure I am paying attention, can hear you, and there's no disruptive background noise or motion.

Be patient and understanding; don't rush, give me time.

Treat me with dignity, respect and empathy.

Respect and empathy are very important.

Don't patronize me.

When I come in to see you, what often happens? You look at my notes and see that I have dementia. Now I have suddenly become the invisible woman!

Please talk to *me*, not my carer, family member or friend. Don't assume I am a mindless empty shell. I am not deaf, and I am there in the room with you. Of course, I might well indicate to you that I would like my supporter to talk on my behalf, so please include them in the conversation, but make sure I am part of this circle of discussion.

Make eye contact with me and use simple clear language. Make sure that I am paying attention, can hear you, and that there's no disruptive background noise or motion around us. Be patient and understanding, as it may take a little longer for me to process information. Don't rush me; give me time to speak. Treat me with dignity, respect and empathy, even if I am having difficulty communicating clearly or understanding you.

> I'm still a human being like you, so don't patronize me. I may well indeed have been a clinician once too, so don't assume anything!

I'm still a human being like you, so don't patronize me. I may well indeed have been a clinician once too, so don't assume anything!

Your stereotype of me!

Don't question my diagnosis – this is what dementia looks like!

Traumatic diagnosis with terminal condition with no cure.

Be sympathetic – symptoms not obvious.

You can't see my enormous inner struggles to cope.

Listen to me and don't minimize my feelings.

I'm an expert in the lived experience of dementia.

And please don't ever question my diagnosis, assuming I have to fit some preconceived stereotype of yours as to what a person with dementia should look like. This *is* what dementia looks like! The symptoms are not always obvious, but I know that things are very different for me now. I am no longer able to cope as well as I used to. But you can't see my enormous inner struggles to cope.

Listen to me and don't minimize my feelings. I am an expert in the lived experience of dementia, so I can teach you a great deal, if only you would listen carefully to what I am trying to tell you.

> Listen to me and don't minimize my feelings. I am an expert in the lived experience of dementia, so I can teach you a great deal, if only you would listen carefully to what I am trying to tell you.

It has been traumatic enough getting this label of dementia, so please treat me sympathetically, trying to understand what it feels like to be diagnosed with a terminal condition for which there is no cure.

Let's move now from how you talk *to* me, to how you talk *about* me and my condition.

Take care with words

Words can influence my mood and self-esteem, and how others around me think about dementia.

You can increase stigma or discrimination against me.

Accurate, respectful, inclusive, empowering and non-stigmatizing words.

Each person with dementia is unique.

I am not my dementia.

Dementia is not a normal part of ageing, nor is memory loss the only problem.

How you talk about dementia can have a huge impact, not only on my feelings while I am seeing you, but also on how I am treated and viewed within the community. The stigma of having this condition is bad enough, without our clinicians adding to it by the way they speak about dementia.

Your words can influence my mood and self-esteem, having a profound impact on how I am able to cope with this struggle to battle the many problems caused during my decline with dementia. We want to hear a positive message, so use language that focuses on our remaining abilities, not on our many and increasing deficits.

> ...use language that focuses on our remaining abilities, not on our many and increasing deficits.

Your words can also influence how others around me think about dementia, and so increase the chance that I will experience stigma or discrimination. The right language must be accurate, respectful, inclusive, empowering and non-stigmatizing. It should reinforce the fact that everyone with dementia is unique, that there are many forms of dementia, and symptoms may present differently in each one of us.

> Respectful language recognizes that I am not my dementia.

Respectful language recognizes that I am not my dementia. It is also factual and does not reinforce stereotypes or myths about dementia. Dementia is not a normal part of ageing, nor is memory loss the only problem that we have. We also can have difficulties with speaking, planning, problem solving, behaviour, mood and sensory perception.

So what should you do?

Talking about dementia

Don't be afraid to ask, especially people of other cultures.

Say:

- Dementia
- Alzheimer's disease and other forms of dementia
- Form or type of dementia
- Symptoms of dementia

Don't say:

- Dementing illness
- Affliction
- Senile dementia or senility
- Demented or dementing

How would you feel?

When talking about dementia, don't be afraid to ask what words we are comfortable with you using. For example, using the word 'dementia' may not be acceptable to people from other cultures or languages. Seek guidance on this where possible. Certainly in some European languages, 'dementia' means 'madness'.

In most cases we would prefer you talk about dementia, Alzheimer's disease and other forms of dementia, a form of, or type of, dementia, and symptoms of dementia.

> It's awful when you talk about
> dementing illness, an affliction,
> senile dementia, senility and,
> most terrible of all, demented.

How would you feel? Suppose you have just gone to your specialist with a few issues, to be told that you are dementing, or in a few years' time will be demented? Suppose now that you are just 46, like I was, and are told this? Now try to imagine you are told it's senility. This clearly is a term dating back to when it was thought that dementia was a normal part of ageing. What if you are not just talking about dementia, but about people with dementia? Here the words you use are even more important to us.

Talking about people with dementia

Don't call us sufferer, victim, demented person, dement (vacant dement!), afflicted, empty shell, not all there.

Don't say I'm fading away or disappearing.

Don't lump us all together, saying 'they' do this or that.

Don't ever say we are absconders, wanderers, offenders, perpetrators, attention-seekers or even inmates!

These words define us by our condition, and are demeaning and derogatory.

People with dementia, living with dementia, with a diagnosis of dementia.

Maintain our dignity and avoid depersonalizing us.

We are people first and foremost, not our condition, so please don't strip away our humanity by calling us sufferer, victim, demented person, dement (even vacant dement), afflicted, empty shell, not all there. And don't say I'm fading away or disappearing. I will always still be here for as long as I am alive.It's even worse when you talk about us as absconders, wanderers, offenders, attention-seekers, inmates – we are not infants, nor are we criminals, nor are we in jail (although it might feel that way in residential aged care). Don't lump us all together, referring to us as 'they', as this loses sight of our unique individuality.

Please simply call us people with dementia, or a person living with dementia, or people with a diagnosis of dementia.

All these terms – and I am sure you can think of others – define us by our condition, and are demeaning and derogatory.

Please simply call us people with dementia, or a person living with dementia, or people with a diagnosis of dementia. It's not that hard to maintain our dignity and to avoid depersonalizing us.

Now, how about the way you talk to our carer, family or friend?

Talking about carer or supporter

Carers are not living with dementia – only we know what it is like to live with dementia.

Caring for, living alongside or supporting a person with dementia – or living with the impact of dementia.

Paul is my family member, husband, supporter, or carer.

Ask us – I call Paul my 'enabler'!

Talking about caring role – impact of or effect of supporting me – only carer knows what it is like to care for us.

Don't say 'carer burden' or 'burden of caring' – use neutral language – but the carer can talk about their difficulties.

This too can have an enormous impact on us. I get so upset when carers say they are living with dementia. Would my husband Paul say something like that if I had breast cancer? Would he say he was living with cancer? Of course not, as he is living alongside his wife who has dementia. Only I know what it is like to live with dementia. He could say that he is caring for a person with dementia, or supporting a person with dementia, or living with the impact of dementia. And when you talk about Paul, he is my family member, my husband, my supporter and my carer. Simply ask what our preference is – mine is that Paul is my enabler, but that's not on any 'official' documentation!

When you talk about the impact of the caring role, speak of the impact on Paul of supporting me, or the effect of supporting me. Only our carer knows what it is like to care for a person with dementia. Avoid talking about the carer burden or burden of caring as that assumes Paul's entire life is negative, and that I am difficult. Try to use neutral language if possible. Of course, our carer can talk about the difficulties they might experience as a result of caring for us.

What about the impact on us?

Talking about symptoms

Each experiences different symptoms, so the impact will be different.

I'm nicer and more people-focused, rather than totally task-driven, according to former staff!

Speak of the impact on us as disabling, life-changing, challenging or stressful, but not hopeless, unbearable, impossible, tragic or devastating.

Be truthful and realistic, but not negative, disempowering, pessimistic or frightening.

Support us to seek social, physical and cognitive engagement.

Encourage us to remain as positive as possible.

The symptoms we each experience will be different, depending on the cause of the dementia and its progression. So the impact on our lives will be different – and not always negative. I have apparently become nicer and more people-focused, rather than totally task-driven!

Speak of the impact on us as disabling, life-changing, challenging or stressful. Please don't say it's hopeless, unbearable, impossible, tragic or devastating. Be truthful and realistic, but there's no need to be negative, disempowering, pessimistic or frightening.

Certainly, it's truly awful for us in the beginning, but the more support we get to seek out social, physical and cognitive engagement, the better our lives will be. Please encourage us to remain as positive as possible.

One area where language can further label and disable us is the whole question of behavioural changes that might occur.

Talking about behaviour

Behavioural and psychological changes often communicate unmet needs – confusion, pain, boredom or loneliness.

As clinicians, you will talk of BPSD – but talk to us and our families about changed behaviours or expressions of unmet need.

Don't talk about behaviours of concern or challenging or difficult behaviours.

Don't talk about us as difficult, aggressor, obstructive, wetter, poor feeder, vocalizer, sexual disinhibitor, nocturnal, screamer, or even violent offender.

Changed behaviour caused by changes to the brain, affected by the environment, health and medication.

I'm always a person first.

Certainly most of us will experience behavioural and psychological changes. But often these are a way to communicate to you our unmet needs, expressing confusion, pain, boredom or loneliness.

As clinicians, you will talk of behavioural and psychological symptoms of dementia (BPSD), but remember these can be spoken of to us and our families as changed behaviours or expressions of unmet need. But please don't call them behaviours of concern or, more dreadful, challenging or difficult behaviours. In the same way, don't talk about us as difficult, aggressor, obstructive, wetter, poor feeder, vocalizer, sexual disinhibitor, nocturnal, screamer, or even violent offender. It should be obvious why not. Our behaviour is caused by changes to our brain and can also be affected by our environment, health and medication.

I am sure you can think of some other real 'doozies',[2] but think about how you would feel if they were applied to you. Despite our symptoms, we are always a person first.

A few other issues about terminology include how you talk about dementia in a research or medical context.

---

2   Australian slang for dreadfully mistaken words or phrases.

Talking clinically

Dementia is a condition, giving rise to set of symptoms resulting from many different types of disease or illness.

When talking about dementia diagnosed under the age of 65, say younger-onset dementia, not pre-senile dementia, as that's outdated.

Not early-onset dementia, as this implies early-stage dementia.

Please don't reduce us to initials – PWD or PWYOD.

We are people with dementia.

Put our personhood first.

Dementia is strictly a condition, not an illness or disease. This is because dementia is exhibited as a set of symptoms which result from many different types of disease or illness.

Also, when talking about dementia diagnosed under the age of 65, this is referred to as younger-onset dementia – definitely not pre-senile dementia, as that's an outdated term. Also the term early-onset dementia is no longer used, as this can be confused with the concept of early-stage dementia.

Please don't reduce us to initials, such as PWD or PWYOD, as it is not good to be just an abbreviation. We are people with dementia. You see, this puts our personhood first.

So how would I try to summarize all of this?

Our preferences

Talking about dementia:
Dementia, Alzheimer's disease,
a form or type of dementia

NOT dementing illness,
demented, affliction, senile
dementia, senility

Talking about us: Person/
people with/living with/with a
diagnosis of dementia

NOT sufferer, victim, dement/
demented, afflicted, offender,
absconder, attention-seeker

**Talking about carers and
supporters:** Living alongside/
with/caring for/supporting a
person with dementia, family
member, carer

NOT person living with
dementia, carer burden, burden
of care

Let's reflect on our preferences, as people with dementia. When you are talking about dementia, we would like you to use the words dementia, Alzheimer's disease, a form or type of dementia. Please don't upset us with words such as dementing illness or senility.

When you are talking about us, we want to be spoken of as a person (or people) with dementia, or who is living with dementia, or who has a diagnosis of dementia. Don't demean us by words such as victim, dement, afflicted, attention-seeker and so on. And don't forget to talk to us, not our carer. Remember we are not invisible or deaf, so include us in your conversation.

When you are talking about our carers and supporters, they are living alongside us or with us, caring for or supporting us. They are living with the impact of dementia, and preferably should be spoken of in the context of their relationship to us – husband, wife, daughter, etc. Please don't say they are living with dementia – only we know what that is like. Avoid the negative connotations of words such as carer burden, although our carer might want to share with you some of their feelings, out of our earshot.

A wrap-up now of a few ways to talk about clinical terminology.

Preferences in clinical context

Talking about impact of dementia: Disabling, challenging, life-changing or stressful

NOT hopeless or devastating

Talking about symptoms of dementia: Changed behaviour, expression of unmet need

NOT behaviours of concern, challenging or difficult behaviours

Talking about dementia: Condition or set of symptoms

NOT illness or disease

When you are talking about the impact of dementia, speak of it being disabling, challenging, life-changing or stressful. Don't drag us down by words such as 'hopeless' or 'devastating'. When you describe the symptoms of dementia, talk of the impact a particular symptom is having.

Then, of course, there are the behavioural and psychological symptoms of dementia. Talk of these as being changed behaviours and expressions of unmet need. Please don't make it all so negative by talking about behaviours of concern, or challenging and difficult behaviours. Remember, dementia is a condition, or a set of symptoms that could arise from a number of different illnesses or diseases.

> There is so much you can change in our lives simply by taking care about how you speak to us and about us.

It might seem like too much to think about or remember, but it's really very easy. Imagine it's you who's being talked to and about. What words would you prefer?

I do hope this brief overview has been of some help. I have some pamphlets here from Alzheimer's Australia for you to take away and refer to. One is called Talk2Me, so speaks of how you should talk to us. The other is the Dementia Language Guidelines, which cover all the areas of talking about dementia, the carer or supporter, and the symptoms of dementia.[3]

Thank you for inviting me to speak to you this afternoon.

---

3   Similar resources are available at www.fightdementia.org.au.

16

There has to be a better way!

Christine Bryden

November 2014[1]

I am really pleased to have been invited to speak at this launch of resources to improve acute care of patients with cognitive impairment.

My name is Christine Bryden, author and advocate for people with dementia. As a person diagnosed with dementia, I am very grateful for the work of the Commission. It has directed its expertise towards improving our lives, particularly drawing attention to the need to improve our hospital experience. I want to describe some of the issues that we face, and how hard it can be for our families.

But why should I speak at this event which is focused on hearing from experts on the issue of people with dementia in hospitals?

---

1   This talk was given as part of the launch of new clinical resources prepared by the Australian Commission on Quality and Safety in Health Care, in Sydney in November 2014. The Commission will develop a clinical care standard to support the implementation of this resource.

Expert in lived experience of dementia

Formerly S&T advisor to PM.

Diagnosed at age 46.

New life in slow lane of dementia.

Know what it feels like to struggle in your world, while disappearing into ours.

I am also an expert – but in the lived experience of dementia. I have been diagnosed, by one of the world's foremost specialists, with dementia. My words are disappearing, my behaviour is no longer calm, cool and collected, and my memory is erratic. There is no way I could manage my former position as science and technology advisor to the Prime Minister. Indeed, it is hard to manage a simple day at home without the support and encouragement of my enabler, my husband, Paul.

Together with all of my friends with the many diseases that cause dementia, I want you to try to understand how hard it is to live in this unusual and very different land. Each day can bring new challenges and losses.

We know what it feels like each day to struggle to cope in your world, while we are disappearing into ours. And our struggle is particularly hard – both for us and our family – when we go into hospital.

I have been hospitalized a few times in recent years, each time staying in for longer than expected. I'll mention my most recent experience, which was last year.

No one here knows I have dementia!

Rushed through emergency confused and distressed.

Wake up in ward – where am I and why?

No coding for my anti-dementia medication.

No anti-dementia medication, no extra care, no staff support.

WHY IS THIS SO?

I was rushed by ambulance to the resuscitation bay in the hospital, and immediately doctors were trying to stabilize my condition. There was a rapid fire of questions, but Paul was still on his way there. I needed him by my side, as I felt very muddled and in pain. By the time I got to the ward, the nightmare became even more vivid. Paul had to leave, and there was no medication written up for my dementia, nor any extra help for me when he was not there. If he had not given me my anti-dementia medication each morning, I would have become more and more confused, and increasingly distressed and unable to cope.

The fact that I had a pre-existing diagnosis of dementia was not recorded anywhere. There was no coding for this, nor screening done. So there was no extra support for ward staff and no explanation in my notes as to why I might have appeared confused. How do we really know how many people with dementia are in our hospitals, when we don't record this reliably? How likely is it that my primary reason for going into hospital will be my dementia? Surely a medical or orthopaedic emergency is more likely. And, of course, there was no identifier in my notes or even by my bed, to alert staff to my needs.

As Julius Sumner Miller has said, 'Why is this so?' when we have coding and resultant extra care available for people with diabetes, estimated to be only 11 per cent of patients, compared with maybe up to 30 per cent with cognitive impairment.[2]

But let's clear up some terminology here, as it is very important to us.

---

2 Julius Sumner Miller (17 May 1909–14 April 1987) was an American physicist and TV personality, best known in North America and Australia for popular science shows, and for asking: 'Why is this so?'

Terminology

Cognitive impairment – not dementia (unless pre-existing diagnosis).

Flag our risk of delirium.

Refer for assessment of dementia.

Don't label us with dementia.

Let's distinguish clearly between cognitive impairment and dementia. It's very important to identify our cognitive impairment, so that our notes can be flagged for an increased risk of delirium. But neither the emergency department nor our initial time in the confusing ward is the place to diagnose dementia.

Of course, if we do have a pre-existing diagnosis of dementia, then that should be on our notes and highlighted for delirium risk. By all means refer us for further assessment and possible diagnosis of dementia, preferably after discharge, or once we have been stabilized on the ward.

I would never want a label of dementia put on me during my confusing and traumatic experience of acute care, as then I would fear being discharged directly into residential care

Now I want to highlight just a few of the issues that we face once we reach the ward.

What is it like?

At night people calling out, where are they and why.

Doctors asking did you have your test yesterday? How would I know!

Did I sign that consent form?

Exhausting daily complex neuropsychological tests!

THERE HAS TO BE A BETTER WAY.

At night I hear people calling out for their wife to take them home. The night staff are stressed out, but so is the person, very confused as to where they are and why. Our routine is upset and our sleep disturbed.

Paul tries to get there first thing in the morning, so he's with me during my waking hours. But often the doctors are there even earlier, on their rounds, asking questions such as 'Did you have your test yesterday?' How am I supposed to know, unless a helpful nurse is at hand to check my file?

Then there is a form to sign, handed to me by a strange person. Later the doctor asks Paul, 'Has she signed a consent form for the procedure?' I have no idea. Only when my file is checked do they realize that I have signed it already. Was this really informed consent? And don't get me started on those exhausting daily complex neuropsychological tests! A pencil and piece of paper is put on my table. Carefully looking at it, I see it is a mystifying way of finding out what I would like to eat tomorrow! I give up, as it is too hard to work out what it all really means. And then a meal arrives, with all its complicated packaging. Without Paul's help, it was too hard to undo everything.

When I was taken for tests, I got lost trying to find the toilet and then my way back. Even in the ward, I was so stressed trying to walk around and then find my way back to my room, as all the rooms looked the same.

So many issues!

Nobody believes me! Or we're placed with frail older people, and are scolded for 'wandering'.

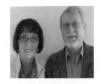

Left alone in strange places waiting for tests, with doctors asking questions.

Trying to cope with way-finding, noise, bustle and confusion, as well as with complicated discharge procedures.

Paul's role in enabling me not acknowledged – his views not sought, nor was he included in consultations with doctors, nutritionists and pain management team.

On the ward, so often I was simply not believed, as I don't look as if I have dementia. This often happens to younger people, as we don't fit your stereotype of a frail older person in late stages. But if we are believed, then we are put with these frail elderly, and there is often no common room to make coffee or watch TV, and we're told off for 'wandering'. But we are simply going for a short walk, even if we get lost due to inadequate signage.

Being in hospital makes our struggles with dementia so much worse! We are left alone in strange places waiting for tests, with doctors, to answer questions, and we are assumed to be totally capable of coping with noise, bustle and confusion, as well as with complicated discharge procedures.

Paul's role in enabling me to cope was not acknowledged, and yet unless he had insisted on being there from 7am till 6pm, it would have been truly awful. His views were not sought, and he was not included in consultations with doctors, nutritionists and the pain management team. It was so hard for me to cope without him at those times when he simply could not be present.

It is so important for us to have our family or friends present for much of the day. And what if we are alone? Could we think of trained volunteers to help us?

Let's look at other issues that occur, even if – or especially when – our diagnosis of dementia is known and accepted.

Why am I treated differently?

I become invisible – people talk about me as if I'm not there.

Watched for BPSD – but these are a way of communicating.

Even physically or chemically restrained – put at risk of harm.

Less chance of rehab or resuscitation.

Why should my disability deny me treatment?

We suddenly become invisible. Everyone talks about us as if we are deaf or simply not in the room! Those dreadful words 'demented' or 'dementing' are even used.

Everything we do in response to the traumatic and confusing environment is simply put down to behavioural and psychological symptoms of dementia (BPSD). But these behaviours are often our only way of communicating to you the issues that we are experiencing – pain, confusion, delirium, feeling alone and lost in an unfamiliar place without our family present.

And even more frightening is that we may be restrained, chemically or physically. This only makes everything so much worse – and places us at risk of harm.

And we may not get adequate treatment – for example, from allied health and rehab. It seems to be assumed that we are beyond help and hope, and not worth the effort. I know that my daughter, who is an acute care cardiovascular physiotherapist, has said that I shouldn't disclose my diagnosis in hospital; otherwise, I might not be resuscitated, might not get good physiotherapy, nor get referrals for ongoing treatment. That's a terrible indictment of our hospital system. Why should my disability deny me treatment?

I'd like to summarize some issues now.

Invaluable for improving our care

Dementia nurse specialist for advice, training and support of nurses, clinicians, porters, cleaners, admin and kitchen staff.

Cognitive assessment or diagnosis coded, delirium risk noted.

Enabling hospital environment, and supporters by our side.

Minimize risk of adverse outcomes, complications, length of stay and readmissions – reducing cost of care and staff stress.

Good for us and for management

Our hospitals have many more people with a cognitive impairment than, say, diabetes, but usually have only diabetes nurse specialists and no dementia nurse specialists. So there's no one staff can turn to for advice, training and support in managing us when we land up in their wards. And it is not just nurses, but clinicians, porters, cleaners, admin and kitchen staff who need to be able to help us. It's not only while we are on the ward that we face problems, but in outpatient departments, having tests and being admitted or discharged.

Those of us with a pre-existing diagnosis often find that our care is not appropriate for our special needs, as this is not coded, and there is no flag on our file or an identifier for some of the issues we might face such as an increased risk of delirium.

The enabling hospital should allow our supporters to assist us, and minimize noise, have good signage and be designed according to dementia-enabling principles.

While in acute care, it is important to minimize the risk of adverse outcomes and complication, as well as reduce length of stay and number of readmissions. Not only is this good for us, but it is also good for management, reducing the cost of our care, and minimizing staff stress.

These new comprehensive and very impressive resources will be a valuable tool for improving our care during any hospital stay by addressing the many challenges that we face. I can't say that I look forward to my next hospitalization, but I am sure it will be a better experience as the result of these resources.

Thank you.

17

Come dance with me!

Christine Bryden

November 2014[1]

I want to introduce you to an exciting dance program in Brisbane for people with dementia. It's called Come Dance with Me.

It was inspired as a result of my appearance on the ABC TV program *Australian Story*,[2] where I was trying to learn to dance with a group of other mature women. I found this class very hard, so I soon gave up, but Bev Giles, Tiina Alinen and Alzheimer's Australia Queensland worked hard to set up a dance class especially designed for people with dementia.

Dance is an activity that we can share with family and friends, bringing joy, fun and laughter. Movement to music, as a creative, physical and social activity, has positive body and brain health benefits for all of us. It enhances visual-spatial memory, sensory experience and emotions, as well as procedural memory. It assists short-term memory and improves mobility and balance.

In this talk I will briefly describe some of the important elements of this program, which make it particularly appropriate for us. As a person living with dementia, I hope that I can give you some unique insights into creative dance.

---

1   Christine has been involved in developing a program of creative dance for people with dementia, and was invited to address the 6th International Arts and Health Conference in Melbourne, November 2014.

2   *Australian Story* is one of the Australian Broadcasting Commission's flagship programs, with a viewing audience over 1 million. The episode was broadcast on 30 June 2015, and rebroadcast four times over the following six months (www.abc.net.au/austory/specials/forgetmenot/default.htm).

About the program

Come Dance with Me is a new dementia-friendly dance program designed to empower people with dementia to participate in their community while engaging in fun, social and physical activity.

When

The next program will start on Thursday 6 November and will run from 10am to 12pm every Thursday for six weeks, ending 11 December.

Where

Newmarket, Brisbane.

Who should attend?

The program is open to people with dementia, their family and friends.

What do I need to bring to the class?

Come Dance with Me was launched as part of Dementia Awareness Month this year. The weekly class is designed to empower people with dementia to participate in their community while engaging in social and physical activity.

The program is open to anyone living with dementia, and our family and friends. Each class is easy to follow and caters for all ages and ability levels. There are no dance steps to remember, no remembering left or right, and no experience in dance is needed – just a willingness to enjoy yourself.

Creative dance offers experiences that can reveal our inner self. Using movement as the communication tool, we are given encouragement to explore ways to express ourselves. There is no wrong way – only our way.

We dance to our favourite music, whether that's Bing Crosby, Louis Armstrong or a movie theme. By using the tools of improvisation, touch, music, tactile materials, voice and movement, creative dance opens up a world of 'in the moment' physical and emotional experiences.

Creating a dementia-friendly society!

'It's wonderful! It's exhilarating! I like the exercise and I love all the beautiful treasures here!'

Our faces are usually sad or anxious to start with, but we leave with a big smiley face!

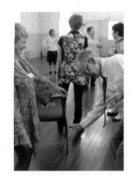

Giving us the opportunity to dance regardless of having dementia is an important part of the national goal of creating a dementia-friendly community. The program is non-verbal, allowing us to enjoy an activity without feeling overwhelmed or outpaced, as so often occurs in other social settings.

One fellow said, 'It's wonderful! It's exhilarating! I like the exercise and I love all the beautiful treasures here!' He loves to dance with the ladies, and his face lights up and he focuses on his partner as if there is no one else in the room.

The feedback forms are simple, just a line of sad and happy faces. Our faces are usually sad or anxious to start with, but we leave with a big smiley face! Feedback so far shows the program has been a great success for people with dementia. So let's look at why this might be so. How can you design a program for us?

No wrong way to dance

It's not what you say, but how you say it!

'I like being creative and moving to the music. I love the bits where we act and can be funny. My anxiety is high at the start, but by the end of it I feel on top of the world.'

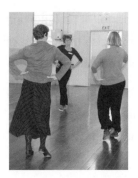

Most importantly, there is no wrong way to dance. Not only does our dance teacher say this, but everything she does affirms it.

People with dementia are very sensitive to emotions and we read people very easily. So even if you say there is no wrong way, but your face or body language says otherwise, then your actual words are meaningless. It's not what you say, but how you say it!

One lady said, 'I like being creative and moving to the music. I love the bits where we act and can be funny. My anxiety is high at the start, but by the end of it I feel on top of the world.'

It's all about moving to the music and having fun, and responding to a dance program that is full of creative ideas.

Tiina Alinen

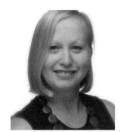

'I enjoy watching participants lose themselves in their dancing. Personalities come out to play in an environment where everything is possible. Seeing faces, especially eyes, come alive when their movement ideas are embraced, is a joy to watch. The infectious laughter within the group keeps the rhythm of the class humming along...I feel very privileged to witness this.'

Tiina Alinen, who brings to the classes her creativity and a welcoming approach to people with dementia, facilitates the weekly classes. She has 30 years' experience in community, creative and professional dance. Her purpose is to value people and connect through the language of movement and dance. She shares her creativity, passion and joy, and reaches out to people with dementia with compassion and warmth. She says:

> I enjoy watching participants lose themselves in their dancing. Personalities come out to play in an environment where everything is possible. Seeing faces, especially eyes come alive when their movement ideas are embraced, is a joy to watch. The infectious laughter within the group keeps the rhythm of the class humming along.

Tiina stresses that:

> The beauty of creative dance is how it embraces inclusivity and how the movement language comes from the participants. What I love the most about these workshops is watching people reveal who they are through their dancing. I feel very privileged to witness this.

Bev Giles

'One of the happiest sights I've ever seen... You seemed so full of mischief and were obviously having a wonderfully carefree time whirling around without a care in the world. That was fantastic.'

'To see you all brimming over with playfulness, exuding joy and creativity and free for that time, at least from the burden of living with dementia. That is what it is all about.'

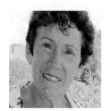

The class has been developed in collaboration with Beverley Giles, who brings more than 25 years' experience working with us. She said:

> I'm already seeing what I have wanted for people living with dementia ever since I discovered what the arts, particularly dance, had to offer. To see you all brimming over with playfulness, exuding joy and creativity and free for that time, at least from the burden of living with dementia. That is what it is all about.

Bev said she felt privileged to be part of the Come Dance with Me community, and valued the friendships made and the experiences shared very highly. She said:

> One of the happiest sights I've ever seen was the week before last. You seemed so full of mischief and were obviously having a wonderfully carefree time whirling around without a care in the world. That was fantastic.

Earlier this year, Bev travelled to the UK to find out more about what creative dance has to offer. She met some very talented teachers, danced with delightful people and shared lots of fun occasions. She did not then, or during any of her previous research, see or experience anything better than what Tiina is sharing with the group and can't wait to see what she has in store for the next sessions.

Free to be ourselves!

'I would not normally do this sort of thing. So it is a bit confronting and challenging. I get a bit emotional about being able just to be me and not worried about what others think. But it feels really great to be OK just being me.'

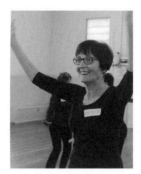

A lady who has been living alone with dementia for a few years said:

> I would not normally do this sort of thing. So it is a bit confronting and challenging. I get a bit emotional about being able just to be me and not worried about what others think. But it feels really great to be OK just being me.

Another lady creates humour in her dance, and is praised for her ability as an actress. You can see her face light up with this affirmation that she has skills of value to the rest of us, after months of feeling loss and grief, and of having felt she was no longer of value in society.

Let's take you through the types of things we do.

Mirroring creates non-verbal conversation

Taking turns to lead and to copy movement, so have non-verbal communication.

In expressive dance, and with mirroring, we participate on equal basis.

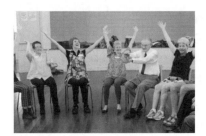

We start with a warm-up, sitting around in chairs. We mirror the leader and take turns as leader. So the movement may be waving our arms or fingers, moving our legs, making a face, even shouting or breathing out loudly. Anything goes!

When we start moving around the room, some chairs stay in the dance space for those of us with balance problems or who need to sit for a while. Mirroring is an important part of what we do, even as we move around the room in pairs or all following the one person. It's all about moving to the music and having a non-verbal conversation in our dance expression. This is why mirroring is so important. We copy movement to create a conversation, and because we are taking turns to lead, this means we are having a non-verbal communication. This puts us on the same footing as you.

All too often in most social settings, we feel overwhelmed and outpaced by the flow of words. Even our thoughts feel shattered by this onslaught, and we drift away, unable to join in at such a fast cognitive pace. Dance that uses words such as left, right or first position, and is focused on remembering steps, disempowers us.

In expressive dance, and with mirroring, we can join in on an equal basis.

What freedom and fun we were having!

One theme was use of coloured scarves.

Blokes preferred sports theme and danced game of cricket!

Another theme was colour, with props (green bucket, red teapot, blue shawl and huge strip of yellow material).

One theme was the use of coloured scarves, and even the blokes were able to find ways to be creative with these. Mind you, they far preferred the sports theme, and acted out – or danced – a game of cricket! Another theme was colour, with props including a green bucket, a red teapot, a blue shawl and a huge strip of yellow material.

I teamed up with another lady with dementia and our theme was green. We moved to the music, planting seeds, watering them with the green bucket, and then growing up to become tall waving willow trees. Then all around us were green meadows, through which we skipped till returning to our waving willow tree. We could vividly imagine ourselves in each of these situations, and we could really feel the colour green.

The huge strip of yellow material became a waving sea under which we could move. Then it was stretched tight so we could push body parts and faces up against it to wonder at the shapes created.

Blue was expressed by slumped shoulders and a downward expression, but also by lifting our hands to the blue sky, and waving our hands down low to create waves in the sea. Red became cherries, fire and flame. Each colour was a chance to move and to create expressions, shapes and actions. We felt encouraged to move to music, and free to create anything that came to mind. What freedom and fun we were having!

Socializing important for keeping brain healthy and to avoid isolation

Withdrawal from society leads to further depression, on top of what we feel because of dismal prognosis.

'I tend to forget to eat. The break is a good reminder. I get quite hot too, so this break gives me a chance to cool down, as there's a nice breeze coming in.'

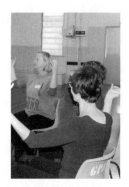

After about an hour of warm-up and dance, we stop for a break. Water, tea, coffee, fruit, cheese and cake are laid out on a table off the main dance area, and we sit around and socialize. This is a very important part of keeping our brains healthy.

Isolation is often a result of our life with dementia. Your friends and family don't keep contact as much as they did, as they don't know what to say or what to do. So we talk less and withdraw from society. This leads to further depression, on top of what we already have because of our dismal prognosis. Dementia is terminal and there is no cure. Depression is only natural, but it makes everything worse.

We forget how to socialize and how to chat. But we often also forget to eat or drink, especially if we live alone. So the break is a key part of our dance class. One lady said that the break is great: 'I tend to forget to eat, so it's a good reminder. I get quite hot too, so this break gives me a chance cool down, as there's a nice breeze coming in.' She really enjoys chatting and laughing over this tea break.

Creating smiley faces

Thank you for participating in the 'Come Dance with Me' program!

Pre-session

Please indicate by ticking or circling how you are feeling at this moment:

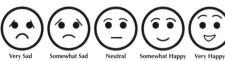

Post-session

Please indicate by ticking or circling how you are feeling at this moment:

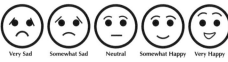

Come Dance with Me is empowering us to participate in a dance program on an equal basis. No longer are we being outpaced and out-talked! Nor are we puzzled by left or right, or the use of lots of words. Instead, we are moving to music and creating ways to express ourselves in non-verbal conversation. We are socializing and remaining active, so our brains are being reinvigorated.

I'd like to thank Alzheimer's Australia Queensland for getting this program up and running. Particular thanks must go to the wonderful Bev Giles, who picked up the pieces after my *Australian Story*, and worked so hard to turn Come Dance with Me into a reality. Thanks also to the lovely Tiina Alinen, whose body language really says there is no wrong way to dance.

I'd like to encourage you all to think about this model for dance with people who have cognitive difficulties. We need your help to dance freely and to express ourselves non-verbally. It's good for us to dance and socialize, as it energizes our brain. Please help make our sad faces into smiley faces!

Thank you.

18

Lisa and I

Christine Bryden

February 2015[1]

I first met Lisa Genova on the internet, back in 2001. I was a founding member of the Dementia Advocacy Support Network International, set up by and for people with dementia.

Lisa had heard about us and asked to join us in our chat room so that she could research her new book. She was a Harvard-trained neuroscientist and this was to be her very first book. We shared our experiences with her, and she read my first book, *Who will I be when I die?* What she says in her book's introduction is that we taught her so much through our intelligence, humour, empathy, willingness to share what was individually vulnerable, scary, hopeful and informative. She said her portrayal of Alice is richer and more human because of our stories.

I am so pleased that many of us who originally chatted with her are still here, still speaking out, and we are all absolutely delighted that Lisa has written a story that is so very powerful and poignant, reaching a huge audience. At first she sold the book out of the boot of her car, until Simon and Schuster published the book in 2009 – and now it is a best-seller around the world! I was thinking about Lisa when I reread the book, this time as an e-book, and emailed her to let her know I was still very much alive, even though now it was 2011.

---

1   This talk was given to an audience in February 2015, before a private showing of the movie *Still Alice*, based on Lisa Genova's best-selling book, arranged by Alzheimer's Australia (QLD) for an audience of people with dementia and their families. Julianne Moore won an Oscar for her part in the film. Lisa sought advice and comment from many members of DASNI in her research. Her book kindly acknowledges Christine and many others from DASNI.

Meeting Lisa here!

Thank you for all you are and do – you are an inspiration!

You are more than what you remember.

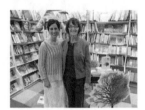

I got an ecstatic email back saying she was in Sydney doing book readings and had only just been talking about our group and also mentioned my name. The very next day she was due to do another book reading here in Brisbane. And that is when I met her, in August 2011, and this picture was taken. After her book reading, we strolled across to Southbank for coffee and chatting for a few hours. She wrote in my copy of *Still Alice*: 'You are more than what you remember' and 'Thank you for all that you are and do – you are an inspiration.'

Lisa is a lovely lady. Not only is she a neuroscientist, but she is an actress, so she literally acts out parts of her books so as to capture them in words. By all accounts the movie will demonstrate how successful she has been. I have kept up to date with her through being friends on Facebook, and her life is now full of red-carpet appearances, and being involved with the production of the movie. She hinted at this movie back in 2011. But by then she was already deep into her next books, which are as equally engaging, about other neurological conditions. So keep an eye out for these, which include *Left Neglected* and *Love Anthony*.

But now let's all sit back and be moved by Alice's story.

19

Dementia – an interesting ride!

Christine Bryden

February 2015[1]

I'm going to give you a bit of background about me, so that this gives you an idea of what drives me now, and what I try to draw on in keeping my brain active. Then I'll describe some of the ups and downs of my journey living with a diagnosis of dementia, to encourage you that even if things seem to look bleak, they might improve. For me, living with a diagnosis of dementia has been a bumpy but interesting ride!

I was diagnosed 20 years ago this May – so I am setting some sort of record for survival. I hope that this in itself can give as many people as possible some hope, for a future in which they might be living with dementia.

After talking a bit about my background, then my journey with dementia, I will talk about what you can do to stay well and live well. Finally, I'll speak about my current efforts and my hopes for the coming years. My overall message to you all is to live well and to stay positive. It is never too late to do all that you can to prevent dementia, or prevent further cognitive decline. There is a lot you can do, and it can be simple and fun.

---

1   Talk given in February 2015, as part of a seminar on dementia research arranged by Anglican Retirement Villages (ARV) in Sydney. ARV is a significant provider of aged care in NSW. ARV is collaborating with researchers on a number of projects, drawing on its large resident population as participants. Christine was invited to address this seminar for residents on 11 February 2015, adding a consumer perspective to that of medical researchers involved in the research ARV were supporting, and many residents were participating in. The particular focus of this project is curcumin, both as a possible preventative and as possible marker for Alzheimer's (curcumin appears to bind with plaques associated with Alzheimer's and can be detected by examination of the eye).

Science background

Biochemist then science publishing in Holland and UK.

Missed buzz of research, joined CSIRO.

Set up CSIRO Office of Space Science and Applications.

Office of Chief Scientist and Secretary of Australian Science and Technology Council.

Advised PM on S&T, set up PM's Science Council, and $130 million CRC program.

Awarded Public Service Medal for service to S&T.

I was a research scientist for a pharmaceutical company in the UK, before working in scientific publishing in Holland and the UK. By the time I came out here, I missed the buzz of the research environment and joined CSIRO, where I worked for ten years with researchers and the mineral, energy and aerospace industry, on research planning, funding and evaluation.

Those of you who saw the *Australian Story* on ABC TV will also know that I helped to establish the CSIRO Office of Space Science and Applications, and became involved with rockets, launch sites and satellites, particularly remote-sensing technologies. It was a very broad science background, one that saw me in good stead for being appointed to lead the Office of the Chief Scientist and becoming Secretary of the Australian Science and Technology Council. In these roles, I advised the Prime Minister on science and technology, as well as being responsible for the Prime Minister's Science and Engineering Council, and the $130 million Cooperative Research Centres program.

In 1994 I was awarded a Public Service Medal for outstanding service to science and technology, the same year as I was divorced. Life was busy and fulfilling, juggling work with the active lives of my three daughters.

But the following year, my life was to change dramatically.

Life changed in an instant!

Numb with shock!

'You have Alzheimer's disease.'

'You must retire immediately.'

'You cannot hold any position of such responsibility.'

'Go home, get your affairs in order.'

Saw more positive specialist.

Medication to help function.

Chose brain over gut!

I had lots of blinding headaches and what I thought were symptoms of stress: getting thoughts and words muddled in my head, being totally exhausted and overwhelmed, and sometimes even losing my way. I simply couldn't cope with too many things at once, nor could I cope with the blinding headaches, so I went to a lovely GP. She finally sent me for a CT, and later an MRI scan.

It was a sunny clear winter's day in Canberra, and I was sitting in the neurologist's office. I was a busy 46-year-old, anxious to get back to work to chair yet another meeting. He stood with his back to me, holding up the scan to the light box, and said, 'You have Alzheimer's disease. You must retire immediately – you cannot hold any position of such responsibility. Go home and get your affairs in order.'

I was numb with shock! I went on sick leave a few days later and arranged to see another specialist, who confirmed this awful diagnosis. But he was more positive, saying we are all unique and there was medication to help me function a bit better. Even though this early medication was simply terrible to my gut, I chose to have a better brain!

Like one-way signpost to nowhere

- At home with girls nine and 14.
- Coped with church support.
- 20-year-old deferred degree so 14-year-old could live with her.
- Couldn't cope with sibling arguments.
- Took all of my energy just to function each day.

I retreated to home, spent time with my youngest girls, who were only nine and 14. My 20-year-old was in Sydney at uni. So we coped as best we could, with immense support from my church. The next year my eldest daughter deferred her degree to help, and one of the girls lived with her. I simply couldn't cope any more with sibling arguments. It took all of my energy just to function each day. Our lives featured on Channel Nine TV's *A Current Affair* a few times, and it was very much a story of courage in the face of what was seen as a horror future. It felt like a one-way signpost to nowhere. And it got worse.

Anticipatory helplessness

▸ My nine-year-old helped shop, cook, clean, recall school stuff.

▸ Her mum, her hero, declining before her eyes.

▸ Her teachers, friends, parents, did not believe her.

▸ Mothers of children in year 5 did not get Alzheimer's.

▸ She was called a liar and ostracized.

Soon, all too soon, I stopped speaking on the phone to disembodied voices that I couldn't recognize, gave up trying to keep track of our finances, and even stopped driving.

This was hard for my youngest daughter to see – her mum, the only one she felt she had left in the world after the divorce, her hero, was declining. I was becoming less and less functional. It was all I could do to make even the simplest of meals. She was my carer and helped me shop and recall what was needed around the house, as well as what was coming up at school. As a nine-year-old, without any support, this was hard. Her friends, their parents and her teachers did not believe her – mothers of children in her year simply did not get Alzheimer's. She was called a liar for sharing about my diagnosis in her school journal, and was ostracized.

The toxic lie of dementia

Doctor's prognosis:

- ‣ decline for five years till demented
- ‣ die after three years in care.

Hospice in slow motion.

Anticipatory helplessness:

- ‣ anticipated not being able to do things
- ‣ when difficult, gave up.

I believed – we all believed – the toxic lie of dementia. The neurologist had given me the typical medical prognosis: I would decline for five years until I was demented, then die after another three years in a nursing home. It was a self-fulfilling prophecy, and felt like 'hospice in slow motion'. I have reflected on this time and call it anticipatory helplessness. We anticipate not being able to do things because of the prognosis of decline. When life becomes difficult, we give up, as we believe it is a sign of the dementia.

It was a miserable time of decline and hopelessness, until I could thrust off this typical reaction to the devastating prognosis and try to reimagine a brighter future. But I had help to do this.

Positive about life

By the end of 1997, decided to assume that life lay ahead of me, despite diagnosis.

Began studies for Graduate Diploma in Counselling for thesis.

- ‣ People with dementia benefit from counselling and from cognitive behavioural therapy.
- ‣ Revolutionary thinking back then!
- ‣ Graduation featured in ABC 7.30 Report.

I had met my spiritual advisor, Reverend Liz MacKinlay, during the year that I got my diagnosis. She came to meet with me each month, to listen and to pray. She is a gerontological nurse specialist, as well as an Anglican priest, and yet had never spoken with a person with dementia before. She was learning so much about the inside perspective that she encouraged me to write about my experiences.

So I began to write about my fears, and called this first book *Who will I be when I die?*[2] This was my biggest fear, paralyzing my ability to think more positively. But, by the end of 1997, I had begun to decide to assume that a life lay ahead of me, despite this diagnosis.

Amazingly, the book was accepted to be published in mid-1998, and is still being sold in several languages around the world. By the time of its publication, I had also begun studies for a Graduate Diploma in Counselling (my final thesis was published in an international journal[3]).I was suggesting that people with dementia could benefit from counselling and from cognitive behavioural therapy, which was truly revolutionary thinking back then! My graduation featured on the ABC TV 7.30 Report, where the journalist reflected on my being awarded the Public Service Medal, and then coping and re-emerging with studies in therapy for people with dementia.

So much was becoming positive in my life! In mid-1998 I made a decision that was to dramatically change my life, and put it on an even more positive path.

---

2   Christine Bryden (2012) *Who will I be when I die?* London: Jessica Kingsley Publishers (first published 1998).

3   Christine Bryden (2002) 'A person-centred approach to counselling, psychotherapy and rehabilitation of people diagnosed with dementia in the early stages.' *Dementia* 1, 2, 141–156.

New life with Paul

Met and married Paul.
Gave hundreds of talks in Australia and around the world.
International advocacy group by and for people with dementia.
Told ADI London we are not 'mindless empty shells'.
Voted on to ADI Board.
Second book *Dancing with Dementia*.

I was lonely and decided to join an introductions agency. My girls thought maybe I really was succumbing to dementia! I met the lovely Paul. As a former diplomat, he was the ideal complement to my science background, and he encouraged me to continue to speak out as an advocate for people with dementia. A year after we met, we married in an amazing ceremony at my church. So many people came who had never thought I would ever be able to find such joy in my life, let alone live long enough to do so.

With Paul's help as my travel organizer and enabler, I have given hundreds of talks in Australia and around the world. I was a founding board member of the very first international advocacy group set up by and for people with dementia. It was the early days of the internet, and we met online and in chat rooms, even face to face on a farm in Montana. I represented the group in London and argued for acceptance and inclusion by Alzheimer's Disease International (ADI). Only the year before, they had written in an annual report that we were 'mindless empty shells'.

Just a few years later, in 2003, I was voted on to the ADI Board and served for three years, while also continuing to speak out to encourage others. I wrote a second book describing this amazing journey, as well as talking about what it feels like and what you can do to help. I called this second book *Dancing with Dementia*,[4] to indicate the metaphor of how Paul and I adjust to the ever-changing and discordant music of my dementia.

It was not all a dance of joy, though.

---

4   Christine Bryden (2005) *Dancing with Dementia: My Story of Living Positively with Dementia*. London: Jessica Kingsley Publishers.

Down – then up!

Broke back – in Tokyo hospital for three weeks.
Fragile – still in great pain.
Exhausted – unable to continue.
Worried – about youngest daughter 'gone off the rails'.
2006–2010 – very few talks as felt as if candle was sputtering out.
2009 – still frail when middle daughter married.
2011 – finally bounced back, giving talks in Australia and overseas about decade of change I had seen.
2012 – giving talks once more around Australia and Japan.
2013–2014 – still speaking, still feeling positive and energized!

In 2004 in Tokyo, after attending the international conference in Kyoto, along with 4000 others, and launching my second book there, I fell over. I broke my cheek, arm, hip and back, and ended up in a Tokyo hospital – alongside frail, tiny Japanese ladies – for three weeks.

Most of the next year I felt fragile, and struggled to walk with a stick, and was still in great pain. I was feeling exhausted – unable to cope or to put on a cheery face. I was very worried about my youngest daughter, who had gone off the rails when she was 13, and was now really struggling. The impact on her of my diagnosis, decline and then marriage and advocacy was just too much for her to deal with.

I gave no talks in 2005, focusing on my daughter and getting my own strength back. Over the next few years I gave only a few talks, here, in Berlin and Japan, but they all ended on a low note, about wanting to retreat. I said that I felt as if my candle was sputtering out. I was still frail when my middle daughter was married in 2009, as well as in 2010 when we travelled to the UK to visit my mother for her 90th birthday, and later for her funeral.

It was not until 2011 that I finally bounced back, giving talks in Australia and overseas about the decade of change that I had seen. By the next year I was giving lots of talks once more, around Australia and in Japan. This burst of energy has been sustained right through 2013 to 2014. Here I am, many, many talks later, still speaking on a range of topics. And I have increasingly become involved in my earliest passion.

Nothing about us, without us!

Consumer representative. Speaks out on what is most important for people with dementia and their families. Relevance of research into dementia care:

▸ not quality of that research
▸ nor balance of biomedical and dementia care research.

Founding member of Consumer Dementia Research Advocacy Network.
Advisory/Steering Committees $25 million Cognitive Decline Partnership Centre.
Steering Committee of Queensland Statewide Dementia Clinical Network.
Scientific Panel of the Alzheimer's Australia Research Foundation.

This is, of course, scientific research. I was a founding member of the Consumer Dementia Research Advocacy Network in 2010. Since then we have been involved in allocating several million dollars of research funding. As consumer representatives, we look at what research might be most important for people with dementia and their families.

I am also involved as advisor in a number of research projects in the $25 million National Health and Medical Research Council's Cognitive Decline Partnership Centre. Some of these relate to hospital care, so link well with my appointment earlier this year to the Steering Committee of the Queensland Statewide Dementia Clinical Network. Recently I was also appointed as a consumer representative on the Scientific Panel of the Alzheimer's Australia Research Foundation, which includes Professor Ralph Martins.[5]

Way back in 2004, at a talk in Kyoto, I said that there should be nothing about us, without us. The involvement of people with dementia as advisors in research is very much part of this, particularly for research into dementia care, prevention and detection. But we are unlikely to be able to comment on the quality of that research, or the balance of funding between biomedical and dementia care research.

Let's never forget that, despite a focus on dementia care, consumers seek preventative and curative medications for the many diseases that cause dementia. We need to do all we can to support research into these efforts. There is a very important way in which we can help researchers do this work.

---

5   Professor Ralph Martins AO was another speaker on that day – Founding Chair of Ageing and Alzheimer's Disease at Edith Cowan University (in West Australia). Christine was making a polite reference as to how they were connected. AO is Order of Australia, similar to the UK's MBE.

Research subjects

Dr Gillings, G7 World Dementia Envoy:
people with dementia accept more risk to find
cure.

Prof. Henry Brodaty says delay onset by five
years, halve number of cases of dementia.

Prof. Karin Anstey developed Body Brain
Life modules for people to prevent or delay
dementia.

Volunteering to be research subjects is one way to help. I am very impressed to hear of the way this centre is participating in Professor Martins' research. It is so important to do this, as how else will we ever find safe and effective treatments to prevent, detect or cure dementia?

Interestingly, Dr Dennis Gillings, the G7 World Dementia Envoy, who recently visited Australia, said that people who are at risk of having or who already have dementia are willing to accept far higher levels of risk than others. We are much more likely to volunteer as research subjects and accept a level of risk.

I think this is because we know there is no cure and no curative treatment. All we have is medication to help us to function better as we struggle to cope with decline. Indeed, Dr Gillings said a person told him that if the risk was getting cancer, at least there was a cure for that.

Prevention is so important. As Professor Henry Brodaty has said, if we could delay the onset of dementia by five years, we would halve the number of cases of dementia. This would be truly amazing!

Professor Karin Anstey's work in prevention of dementia is looking at ways to increase awareness of the need to have a healthy lifestyle. Her group has developed Body Brain Life modules for people to look at how much they are doing in terms of prevention.

And let's look at what's needed.

5 Steps to brain health

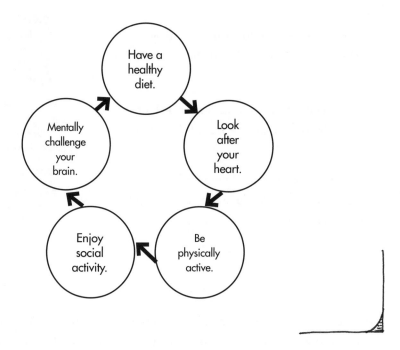

We need to look at our lifestyle, and to start this in middle age if at all possible. But it's never too late to start the five simple steps to brain health: have a healthy diet, look after your heart, be physically active, enjoy social activity, and mentally challenge your brain. I try to eat well and to do around 30 to 40 minutes of moderate exercise five times a week. I take our keen little toy poodle rushing around our neighbourhood most days. Mind you, it's a case of rushing between doggie post-it notes! He sniffs the lamppost to check who has visited and when, leaving him an olfactory message. Then he decides whether or not to mark it himself. Then off we go to the next lamppost or tree!

NOTHING ABOUT US, WITHOUT US!

Steps to brain health

Rush around neighbourhood for 30–40 minutes most days – mostly between doggie 'post-it notes'!

'Never give up, never, never give up, never, never, never give up!'

Continuing efforts such as being a research advisor and giving talks.

We must not forget to remain socially engaged. My mum soon became isolated after my father's death, but perked up when she went into a care home where she could socialize with new friends and take walks in the grounds.

Importantly, we need to mentally challenge our brain, to keep it firing on all cylinders. This brain gym could be playing bridge, golf or the piano, sewing, fishing, gardening – and trying new things wherever possible. For me, it is my passion to become more involved in research advisory roles and to continue my efforts to write and give talks. I have a new book [this book] being released next year.

So focus on healthy eating, physical exercise, socializing and brain activity, and, taking inspiration from Winston Churchill, never give up, never, never give up, never, never, never, give up.[6]

But it need not be a life of misery – of grapefruit, bike-riding, chatting to those you don't like and doing endless crossword puzzles. Let's look at a wonderful example.

---

6   Winston Churchill spoke words similar to these in a speech given to pupils at Harrow School on 29 October 1941: 'Never, never, in nothing great or small, large or petty, never give in except to convictions of honour and good sense. Never yield to force; never yield to the apparently overwhelming might of the enemy' (www.winstonchurchill.org/resources/quotations/quotes-faq).

Jeanne Calment

Took up fencing aged 85.
Rode bicycle till 100.
Lived alone till 110.
Two cigs per day – gave up at 120.
Poured olive oil on food and rubbed it
on to her skin.
Port wine every day, 1kg dark chocolate
per week.
Outlived husband, child and
grandchildren.
Died 122 without dementia.

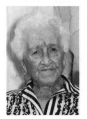

Jeanne Calment lived to be 122, without any sign of dementia.

Let's look at her lifestyle. At age 85, she took up fencing and rode her bike until her 100th birthday. But she was not very athletic, nor was she fanatical about any of this. She lived on her own till just before her 110th birthday, when she had a cooking accident due to failing eyesight. But she carried on walking until she was nearly 115 and broke her femur.

Jeanne smoked two cigarettes a day from the age of 21 to the age of 117, and drank port wine regularly. She even managed to consume nearly a kilo of chocolate each week! That's a lot of chocolate – thank goodness, as I am a committed chocoholic!

What did she say her secret was? She poured olive oil on her food and rubbed it on to her skin. But she said that the main secret was her calm attitude to life: 'That is why they call me Calment.' So choose to be positive, calm and relaxed, to the extent this is possible. It is not always easy for me, so Paul sometimes has his work cut out keeping me calm!

There are two other things besides your attitude that I think make a difference, but, as they are hard to measure, there is often little mention of them.

What more can you do?

Emotional support from family and friends.

Recognize your spiritual self – art, music, nature; for others a form of organized religion.

Nourish your spirit, not just your body.

For me, it's my Christian faith which gives me hope in an eternal future.

Treatment delayed is treatment denied.

The first is emotional support from friends and family if at all possible. This can help us feel less alone as we become more frail or face illness.

The second is recognizing that we have a spiritual side, to give us a different perspective on our life. Make sure that you nourish your spirit, not just your body. For some it could be art, music or nature; for others a form of organized religion. For me, it's my Christian faith which gives me hope in an eternal future.

To have a healthy brain, we need to eat well, look after our heart, be physically active, enjoy social activity and mentally challenge our brain. Also, we should try to be calm, have emotional support and nurture our spiritual self.

But what if, like me, you have been already diagnosed with dementia? Well, I think it's never too late. First of all, make sure that you take the anti-dementia medication without delay. I have always said that treatment delayed is treatment denied, as these medications can slow our functional decline from the point at which we start taking them. The later in our decline that is, the lower the starting point in trying to maintain as much function as possible.

But don't give up. Remember my earlier reference to Churchill? Never, never, never give up.

What else?

Love of family and friends to bring us through emotional lows.

Nurture spiritual self – art, music or nature, organized religion.

Christian faith gives me hope in an eternal future.

We prevent – but what if we have dementia already and want to delay decline?

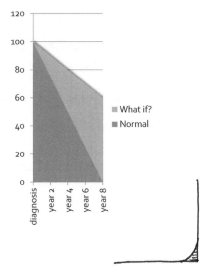

Why should we give up after a diagnosis of dementia? Why should we stop trying to have a healthy brain?

Surely if we can prevent or delay dementia by healthy brain activities, if we continue them after diagnosis, they should also delay or slow down our functional decline.

I've tried to depict what a slowed decline might look like in this imaginary chart. What if we continued preventative measures after our diagnosis? Would that mean we could slow our functional decline, say over eight years, as depicted in lighter grey in my artistic representation. It would be good for there to be research to see if this is possible.

But, in the meantime, I will keep eating well, being physically active, socially engaged and cognitively challenged. I'll also make sure I treasure the love and support of family and friends, as well as nurture my spiritual self.

So what do I hope for the future?

Waiting for cure

Last long enough!
Keep on focusing on brain health.
Learn to type.
Develop research project for evaluating dance program for people with dementia.
Become research advisor in biomedical and psychosocial dementia research.
My scan above, normal below.

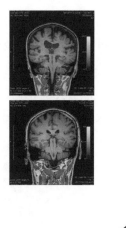

I hope to last long enough to see a cure for whatever is causing the steady disappearance of my brain. I have lasted almost 20 years, but I will probably need to last much longer to see a cure.

My neurologist looked at my latest scans and said clearly I do have considerable connectivity issues. Even the link between the two halves of the brain is thinning. Maybe you can see the difference between my 2011 scan at the top, where grey is brain and black is empty space, and the scan underneath, which is that of a person around the same age, who has a lot more brain than me. And now, of course, my scan in July showed that even more brain has gone.

With determination and effort to prevent functional decline, it may be possible for me to minimize the decline in function despite the ongoing brain damage. I will eat well, look after my heart, exercise, socialize and mentally challenge my brain. I will also treasure my family and friends, and nurture my faith.

For my continued efforts to challenge my brain, I will need to keep on taking on more and more complex activities. These can be simple challenges like learning to type over the next month or so, to more complex ones, based on my science background, such as becoming involved in developing a research project for evaluating the emotional impact of our Come Dance with Me program on people with dementia. I would also like to become involved as a research advisor in a range of other activities, including in the biomedical as well as the psychosocial sciences.

What drives me to keep going and to do all of this?

What keeps me going?

To speak out for all those people with dementia who can no longer speak out.

To talk about what it is like and what you can do to help.

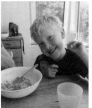

To delight in each one of my grandchildren as they grow older.

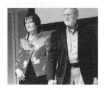

It's my loving husband and enabler, Paul, my daughters and my delightful grandchildren. But also I want to keep speaking out for all those people with dementia who can no longer speak, and to talk about what it is like and what you can do to help.

I hope that what I have said will encourage at least some of you to do whatever you can to prevent dementia. Focus on the five steps to brain health. Don't give up if you have already got a diagnosis. Instead, keep on having a healthy diet, looking after your heart, being physically active, enjoying social activity and mentally challenging your brain.

There's no need to give up hope in a reimagined future at any age. Be encouraged to know that it need not be all doom and gloom! Remember Madame Calment who began fencing at the age of 85, drank port wine and ate heaps of chocolate! Be calm and positive, and relaxed about keeping your brain as healthy as possible.

I congratulate you in being willing to participate in Professor Martins' work. Let's hope researchers will soon find the cures and preventative treatments that we need.

Thank you so much for listening to me.

20

Who was I?
Who am I now?
Who will I be
when I die?

Christine Bryden

May 2015[1]

Who was I?

Twenty years ago I used to be the science and technology advisor to the Australian Prime Minister, responsible for two major advisory councils and for giving the government key advice on a range of policy issues such as genetic engineering, nuclear technology, biotechnology – and the very new internet.

I was recently divorced from my first husband, and somehow managed to juggle my work with being a mother to three girls aged nine, 13 and 19. My life was fulfilling and busy, and a promising future lay ahead of me.

But then all this changed in just half an hour at the neurologist's rooms, when he looked at my MRI scan and test results, and said, 'You have dementia, and must retire immediately. Go home and get your affairs in order.' It is a day fixed in my somewhat broken memory, standing out like the assassination of John Kennedy might do. It was a bright Monday morning on 22 May 1995, and it changed my identity forever. My diagnosis led to the existential questions: 'Who am I now?' and 'Who will I be when I die?'

---

1   The President of the British Psychological Society, Professor Elizabeth Peel, invited Christine to give a talk at a Society Research Seminar, 'Ageing in context: identities and diversities', organized by the University of Worcester Association for Dementia Studies, on 6 May 2015.

Who am I now?

Toxic dementia prescription:

'You have five years till demented, three years till you die.'

No cure or curative treatment.

Who am I now?

Nothing but hopelessness lies ahead.

Hopelessness leads to helplessness.

We give up trying – anticipatory helplessness.

Paralyzed by fear of future loss piled on loss.

Abandon hope all ye who enter here.

On that fateful day 20 years ago, the neurologist gave me what I call the toxic dementia prescription: 'You have around five years till you become demented, then another three years or so in full-time care before you die.' There was no mention of a cure or even of curative treatment, and at that stage no mention even of any symptomatic treatment.

Like the Christian embarking on Dante's journey into the inferno, we fear what lies ahead: 'Abandon hope all ye who enter here.' Who am I now if I can no longer work, be a mother to my children, a friend to others? Who am I now if nothing but hopelessness lies ahead? This hopelessness leads to helplessness. Each time something becomes difficult, we think it's a sign of impending doom and we give up trying. So we experience what I call anticipatory helplessness, believing the toxic dementia prescription, and so fulfilling it with our inaction.

We become paralyzed by the fear of the future, of loss piled upon loss. We fear the stereotype of the end stage of dementia, believing that nothing lies between.

Death in a state of unknowing

Fear of ceasing to be, of losing my selfhood.

How can I face the process of dying – this existential crisis – with dignity?

Will I have any personal resources left within me to deal with it?

From the moment of diagnosis, we are on this journey towards disassembly, losing what we need to face this final battle.

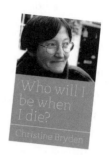

So we face our ultimate fear – of death in a state of unknowing. It's a fear of ceasing to be, of losing selfhood.

Who will I be when I die? My first book has this title[2] and expresses this fear that I had of a total loss of my identity and of being unable to face death with dignity but in a state of disassembly. I felt that I could die of cancer, say, with dignity, but with dementia I feared that I would be unable to face this last battle with any semblance of my own strength and ability.

Death in itself is a loss of identity – the ultimate existential crisis. The process of dying, of facing up to this loss, is one we hope we can face with our own personal resources, our own life story and our own abilities, drawing deep on strengths we might find in our inner being. But when we are diagnosed with dementia, we are not sure what resources will be left to draw on as we undergo this final battle.

Who will we be when we die?

---

2   Christine Bryden (2012) *Who will I be when I die?* London: Jessica Kingsley Publishers (first published 1998).

Only a 'being' label of 'person with dementia'

Exiled from our former self, having lost all our 'doing' labels of family, work and community roles.

We have joined a category of people who are all alike, losing our identity…

And our diversity – only the MMSE now defines us.

But at what stage can you possibly say that I have become like all people with dementia?

**When you have met one person with dementia,
you have met one person with dementia.**

Death lies ahead of us, but our real life lies far behind us. Somehow we have become exiled from our former self. In this experience of exile, we have lost all our 'doing' labels of work and family roles, as well as our own particular community value label.

The only label we have been left with is a 'being' label. We do not *do* anything; we simply exist as people with dementia. Suddenly, we have joined a category of people who are all alike, without any function or role in society.

We have lost not only our identity but also our diversity. Everything that once made us a unique human being, an individual with value to society, has been lost. The only thing that now identifies us is our Mini Mental State Examination (MMSE) score.

But when you have met one person with dementia, you have met one person with dementia. Just like you, we have a rich life story and personality. For at what stage can you possibly say that I have become like all people with dementia? How can you possibly assume that all people with dementia are alike, all sharing only the single 'being' label – of being a person with dementia? How can you possibly reduce us all to an MMSE? How can you strip us of personhood unless you believe that each person with dementia has lost everything that once made us human?

> …when you have met one person with dementia, you have met one person with dementia.

What makes us all human?

'A person is a person through another person.'

'No man is an island, entire of itself. Each is a piece of the continent, a part of the main.'

Do people with dementia share in your humanity? Or are we simply mindless empty shells?

Humans are created to be in relationship with others, to relate and to express our humanity. Without connectedness with others, we lose an important sense of identity – of meaning in life.

And yet people with dementia are often excluded from human relationships.

It is hard to sustain meaningful human interactions when your cognition and communication is failing.

So others must sustain our personhood in relationships with us.

So what is it that does make us human, setting us apart from other mammals? Do people with dementia share in your humanity? Or are we simply mindless empty shells? What is it that makes us all human?

Humans are created to be in relationship with others, to relate and to express our humanity. Without connectedness with others, we lose an important sense of identity – of meaning in life. The Zulu saying captures this: 'A person is a person through another person.' And John Donne wrote: 'No man is an island, entire of itself. Every man is a piece of the continent, a part of the main.'[3] And yet people with dementia are often excluded from human relationships. Others say of us, 'She won't remember I visited,' 'He doesn't make much sense,' 'She never asks about how I am.' These are all devastating statements, as they are all self-centred, assuming that if another person has nothing to give, then they are no longer worthy of human relationship.

Of course, it is hard for us to bring as much to human interaction, so these hurtful comments may often be true. Indeed, it is hard to sustain meaningful human interactions when your cognition and communication are failing, but it is all the more important for others to sustain our personhood in relationships with us.

We are still fully human, worth relating to, but our personhood is so often denied us.

---

3   John Donne (1624) *Devotions upon Emergent Occasions*, Meditation 17.

Look through the lens of an experiential model of dementia

We can be isolated, outpaced, overwhelmed and demeaned by a biomedical model of dementia – my dementia defines me.

See dementia as a shift in my experience of the world – slower to speak and understand, slower to move and react, forgetful of facts and people, impeded in my communication.

Growing chasm between us, created through increasing difference between our cognition and communication. You can bridge this gap to sustain a relationship critical to my personhood.

I AM fully human before our interaction, but when you relate to me, now YOU SEE that I am fully human.

This is the vital difference that YOU have made by bridging the gap between us.

Tom Kitwood's work[4] spoke of the way in which our personhood is damaged by what he calls malignant social psychology. I find that those around us isolate us, outpace us, overwhelm us, demean us, through seeing us only through the lens of the biomedical model of dementia.

We are a diseased person, and our dementia defines us. But you need to look at your interactions with people with dementia through a different lens – of the experiential model of dementia. Dementia, then, is a shift in the way in which I experience the world. I am far more than my dementia. I am a human being, who has a disease of the brain which has an impact on my ability to interact with you.

I am slower to speak and to understand, slower to move and to react, forgetful of facts and of people, and impeded in my communication. These difficulties that I am experiencing mean that there is a growing chasm between us, created through an increasing difference between our cognition and communication abilities. You have the ability to bridge this gap, and to sustain an interpersonal relationship that is critical to my personhood.

I *am* fully human before our interaction, but once you relate to me as best you can, now *you see* that I am. This is the vital difference that you have made by bridging the gap between us.

---

4   Tom Kitwood was a pioneer who tried to understand what care is like from the standpoint of the person with dementia. Published in 1997 by Open University Press, his book *Dementia Reconsidered: The Person Comes First* speaks of harmful care in terms of malignant social psychology.

We share the same human needs

Maslow: Self-actualization is key to a meaningful life
Frankl: Finding meaning to life empowers us
Nietzsche: 'He who has a why to live for can bear with almost any how'
What meaning does our life have?
How can others empower us to find meaning?
Examine how seven domains of wellbeing can help you do this:

Identity	Meaning
Connectedness	Growth
Security	Joy
Autonomy	

As human beings, people with dementia share with you the same needs. Not only do we simply want our basic physical needs met, but, just like you, we seek fulfilment of our higher needs. As early as 1943, Abraham Maslow recognized in his hierarchy of human needs that we all share in the highest need of self-actualization, which he saw as the key to meaningful life.[5]

Concentration camp survivor Viktor Frankl used quotes from philosopher Friedrich Nietzsche to argue that a meaning of life empowers us: 'He who has a *why* to live for can bear with almost any *how*.'[6]

So what is the implication for those of us with a diagnosis of dementia? What meaning does our life have? How can others relate to us in finding meaning? How can we be empowered through finding a meaning in our life?

Dr Al Power, in his latest book *Dementia Beyond Disease*,[7] writes of how we can do this through following seven pathways to wellbeing. He draws on the work of N. Fox *et al.* in 2005[8] to describe these domains of wellbeing: identity, connectedness, security, autonomy, meaning, growth and joy. There will, of course, be as many ways to describe each of these as there are individual people. It seems so obvious to me that none of us is the same, even people with dementia.

---

5   Abraham Maslow's hierarchy of needs is a well-known theory in psychology that he proposed in his paper 'A theory of human motivation' originally published in 1943 in *Psychological Review* 50, 370–396.
6   Friedrich Nietzsche, quoted by Viktor E. Frankl (1985) *Man's Search for Meaning.* New York: Washington Square Press.
7   Power, G.A. (2014) *Dementia Beyond Disease: Enhancing Well-Being.* Baltimore, MD: Health Professions Press.
8   Fox, N., Norton, L., Rashap, A.W., Angelelli, J., *et al.*, (2005) *Well-being: Beyond Quality of Life. Now available as The Eden Alternative Domains of Well-being™: Revolutionizing the Experience of Home by Bringing Well-being to Life.* Available at www.edenalt.org/about-the-eden-alternative/the-eden-alternative-domains-of-well-being, accessed on 3 July 2015.

The first four domains...

Identity: Relate to each one of us as each one of us, not as a labelled people.

Connectedness: Isolation is so often the result of a diagnosis, and yet humans need to be in relationship.

Security: Everything is becoming strange, unknown and unremembered in this unfamiliar territory, where we can be overwhelmed by emotions of the past, a stressful present and an unknown future.

Autonomy: We fear losing our independence, and finally ending up in dementia prison.

Be a care-partner, connect, relate, offer security, soothe our inner struggles and support us through our fears.

There is a hierarchy to these domains, with **identity** being the most important. It rears its ugly head at the moment of diagnosis. It is vital to treat each one of us *as each one of us*, not as a group of people with dementia, nor to label us with such soul-destroying terms as 'dements' or 'absconders'.

Connectedness is essential, as isolation is so often the result of a diagnosis. Fear and embarrassment mean we withdraw, and often we need to be sought out and related to. In so doing you can restore our sense of self. As I said, humans are created to be in relationship.

Security is a challenge for us, when everything is becoming strange, unknown and unremembered. In this unfamiliar territory we can become more emotional and less cognitive. We might become overwhelmed by past emotional baggage, so abuse and stress can rear up unbidden to surround us once more. Past, present and dream can all become mixed up. You will need to do what you can to soothe our inner struggles and to understand these emotional realities.

Autonomy is threatened, as we fear losing our independence – for example, through losing our licence – and finally ending up in dementia prison. Understand these fears and be our care-partner, adjusting your care where we need it, so that we can retain independence for as long as possible.

NOTHING ABOUT US, WITHOUT US!

The final three domains

Meaning: Being stripped of cognition and reliable emotion, maybe we are discovering our true inner self. Help us to connect with whatever once used to give us meaning, such as nature, music, art, religion.

Growth: There is a new future ahead of us within this new prism which is casting such strange beams of light. We can learn how to live a new life in the slow lane of dementia and discover how to simply 'be'.

Joy: By being quietly present with us in the moment and nurturing our senses, we may find moments of joy.

Meaning can be discovered in living in the present moment. We feel stranded in time, with a cloudy idea of the past and no clear sense of the roll-out of future events. But what we do have is an intense experience of the present moment. As we travel this journey from diagnosis to death, being stripped of a cognitive outer self and a reliable emotional self, maybe we are discovering our true inner self, our spirit self. This is where you can help us to find meaning through connecting with whatever once used to give us meaning, such as nature, music, art or religion.

Growth may seem counterintuitive for a person with dementia, especially shortly after diagnosis, but there is a new future ahead of us. We can create what I call a new life in the slow lane of dementia, within this new prism which is casting such strange beams of light. Once we adjust to the changes within us and around us, we learn how to live a new life without our former labels and discover how to simply be.

Joy is perhaps even more challenging to regard as part of wellbeing in dementia, but it will depend very much on those other domains to sustain it. By being quietly present with us in the moment, and nurturing our senses – touch, aroma, vision, taste – you can find moments of joy. Build on the other six domains and find the joy within each person with dementia.

Applying domains in my own life with dementia

Exiled from my identity as a successful working mother, I have a new identity as a dementia advocate.

I do this with the connectedness I have with Paul, who relates to me with love.

Through Paul I have also found security, as he reassures me of his loving presence.

Paul is my enabler, sustaining my autonomy by adjusting his care.

I have found meaning through advocacy and reflections on my spirituality.

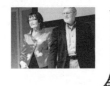

Now I can see growth and have hope for my future.

The way in which these domains build on one another is seen in my own life. I am now exiled from my identity as a mother and in being successful at work, but have found a new identity as an advocate for people with dementia. But I could not do this without the connectedness that I have found with Paul. He relates with love to me, no matter what I might be doing or saying. Through his presence I am connected and fully human. Through Paul I have also found security, as his familiarity is always there, and he reassures me of his loving presence. Paul is my care-partner, my enabler, sustaining my autonomy by adjusting his care so that I can retain independence for as long as possible. I have found meaning in this new life with dementia through my advocacy, through my relationship with Paul and in new reflections on my spirituality.

Life with dementia has been an up-and-down affair, but now I can see growth. I am doing all I can to prevent further decline through remaining physically, socially and mentally active, as well as eating healthily. It's resulting in cognitive, social and spiritual growth.

Joy and wellbeing

Building on these six domains of wellbeing, I have found my way through to moments of joy.

A long 20-year exile from who I once was, to asking who I will be when I die, to knowing now who I am becoming.

Each one of us, with or without dementia, is unique – no one else on this planet shares our identity, but together we form the diversity of humanity.

Even if one day you have dementia, I hope that you will find joy and a sense of meaning, retaining your own identity within this diversity.

By these six domains of wellbeing, I have found my way through to joy. Each moment of the day I can try to discover moments of wellbeing, which together make my day a joyful and fulfilling one. I have heard Professor Julian Hughesspeak of this creation of many moments of wellbeing as being an important way to encourage people with dementia.[9]

Each one of us, whether we have dementia or not, has a need to find meaning in life. But people with dementia need your help to work through the domains of wellbeing, to discover this sense of meaning, and to finally find joy in their lives.

It's been a long 20-year journey of exile, of surviving, and then of thriving. Those words labelling me with dementia changed me from who I once was, to a point of asking who I will be when I die, to knowing now who I am becoming.

Every single person, with or without dementia, is a unique individual. No one else on this planet shares your particular identity. But together we all form the diversity of humanity. You may have dementia, one day, just like me. I hope that you will find joy and a sense of meaning, retaining your own identity within this diversity. We can all benefit from the tremendous changes in perspective that have occurred during the last two decades.

Thank you.

---

9   International dementia expert, Professor Julian Hughes spoke in Australia in 2013, launching his paper 'Models of dementia care: Person-centred, palliative and supportive'. Professor Hughes is a consultant in the psychiatry of old age based at North Tyneside General Hospital, and honorary professor of philosophy of ageing at the Institute for Ageing and Health, Newcastle University. His most recent book is Thinking Through Dementia, published by Oxford University Press in 2011.

21

Pastoral care of people with dementia

Christine Bryden[1]

This morning I'll be giving a talk about my own views about pastoral care for people with dementia.

I'll start my talk with a brief explanation of why I am here. I was diagnosed with dementia in 1995, at the age of 46, and was not expected to last more than about eight years. I'm now 65, and next year it will be 20 years since that awful diagnosis – a miracle that cannot be explained by my doctors!

I believe that I am still here by the grace of God, surviving dementia and doing my best to speak out on behalf of all those who cannot or do not want to speak out for themselves. I believe this is my calling, compelled and enabled by our Lord to reach out and help others understand what it feels like to have dementia and what you can do to help.

I have written two books about my journey, which continue to help people with dementia and their families, as well as professional care-givers and pastoral care workers.

In this talk, I want to try to change your perception of dementia, to see it from the inside out. I hope this might help you in the enormous challenges of pastoral care and ministry to people with dementia.

---

1 Christine has given this talk to many church, chaplaincy, family and community groups, modified as appropriate to the particular audience.

Damage to my brain

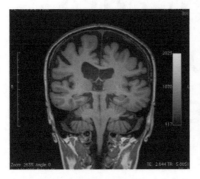

My brain

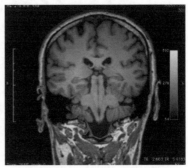

Normal brain

Before I start, I want to show you the damage to my brain, which is so clearly visible on this high-resolution MRI scan. My scan is on the left compared with a normal brain on the right. Given this extensive brain damage, my specialist cannot understand why I can still speak, but I believe God has enabled me to claw my way back from the brink, after several years of increasing disability, to be able to describe what it feels like, and what you can do to help.

Even now, on my bad days I have glimpses of decline and increasing disability, which gives me an authentic empathy and understanding of all those I meet, in Australia and elsewhere, who are struggling each day with dementia. When I visit day, respite or residential care, I can truly empathize with those people with dementia who can no longer speak or function very well at all.

Dementia is the result of around one hundred illnesses which lead to increasing disability and eventually death. Alzheimer's, vascular and Lewy Body dementia are the most common, but for younger people often fronto-temporal dementia is the cause – this is what I have.

So my perspective is through the lens of dementia. We are on a journey towards greater and greater dependency on others, as our communication and other functions decline. It's a journey of increasing need, in which we desperately need your pastoral care and ministry.

A long journey of…

Shock and horror of what lies ahead.

Fear of becoming an empty shell.

Grieving continual and multiple losses.

Dissolution of our being and personality.

Exclusion from society.

Exiled from former self.

**Travelling towards new world of
forgetfulness and confusion.**

It is vital to minister to our spiritual needs, not just our physical and emotional needs, for at what stage on this journey can you say I have become an empty shell? So often the long journey of dementia, of living with dementia each day, facing multiple losses, is ignored. And yet we travel this journey with the fear of the late-stage stereotype of dementia uppermost in our minds. Will our mind become absent and our body an empty shell? When will that happen?

As we face the dissolution of our being, we urgently need ongoing palliative care that affirms our humanity. Each day, we are approaching the end of life, and it is important for us to be helped to reflect, to find a sense of meaning, and for our spirit to be nourished. It is absolutely vital to offer us pastoral care at all stages on our journey, for we face continual and multiple losses and fears, as well as exclusion from society and exile from our former self. Who are we when we have lost all our labels – worker, wife, mother, volunteer, church lay-reader?

Your pastoral care needs to begin at the moment of diagnosis, when we face the shock and horror of what lies ahead. We feel lost, abandoned, without hope, fearful, and questioning of our God. We face years of loss piled upon loss, and a gradual change in who we are in the cognitive world, towards a new world of forgetfulness and confusion.

And, importantly, we are finding it more and more difficult to communicate.

Disease of communication

Slow down, sit quietly, listen and connect.

Watch for non-verbal communication.

Use pauses to give us time to process pictures in our head into gestures, facial expressions or words.

Having dementia significantly impairs our ability to communicate – to form words and to understand. Certainly my capacity to communicate is severely impaired compared with 1995, when I was advising the Prime Minister on Science and Technology. I prepare these talks and read them carefully, rather than speak to brief notes on an enormous range of issues as I once used to do. Even over the past few years, my vocabulary has decreased and the time taken to speak a talk out has increased.[2]

Perhaps we could say that dementia is a disease of communication, creating an unseen barrier between your world and ours? So take time to listen, use pauses to give us time to process what you are saying and how to make the pictures in our head into gestures, facial expressions or words for you to understand. These pauses may feel very odd at first, but they enable us to connect with you. Slow down, sit quietly, listen and connect.

Watch carefully for our non-verbal communication. Remember that everything we do or utter is a way of communicating. So often we are dismissed as simply making meaningless sounds, or just being difficult. We do not have challenging behaviours, simply communicative behaviours – these are often all we have left to relate to you with.

We feel isolated in this fast-paced cognitive world.

---

2   The time that I take to try to read a word, understand it, and then formulate this word in my mouth so as to speak it out, so as I decline it takes me increasingly longer to give a talk.

Outcasts of today's society

Jesus ministered to the lepers.

Reach out to us and overcome your fear.

Untouchables in a world of cognition.

With increasing disability, we need your pastoral care.

We are like outcasts in today's hyper-cognitive society. Like the lepers of Jesus' day – and this lady in Japan whom I met a year or so ago – we need you to touch us, to reach out to us and to bring us spiritual healing.

Seek us out, as we may well have excluded ourselves. We feel like the untouchables of society. Please touch us in our perceived uncleanness and try to see past our very difficult behaviour. Try to overcome your fear of dementia and see past our impeded communication and our limited understanding.

Do not deny us our humanity. For at what stage of my decline can I be denied my selfhood and my spirituality? Surely cognition and emotion are not the only measure of our common humanity? So focus on what connects us, not what separates us.

Our increasing disability urgently needs your pastoral outreach and reassurance that we are in your memories, that you will not forget us on our journey, that you will keep on visiting us and will minister to us as we become more and more dependent on the spiritual care of our Christian fellowship.

So how can you support us and minister to our spirit as we grieve multiple losses and cope with increasing disability? How can you meet the challenge of pastoral care to those with cognitive disabilities?

Bring Christ's love to us

Be alongside, truly present in spirit, and connect without words.

Carry our story and relate to us.

Touch, eye contact, music and aroma can breach the barrier of communication.

Look into our eyes to see the spark that alights when we connect.

Create moments of wellbeing.

Pastoral care of people with dementia is true chaplaincy – it's about 'being alongside'. It's about being with us and connecting with us, without words. Heal us by your presence – bring us peace – as you connect with our spirit deep within.

Try to find out more about us, so that you can help us to find meaning in our lives. Our life story is a springboard for meaningful engagement. You can carry our story for us and relate to us as a whole human being, with dignity and respect. Focus on what we can still do, rather than all the many things we can no longer do. And don't belittle or demean us – we need your understanding, not your fear, derision or embarrassment.

Try to discard temporarily your own masks of cognition and emotion, so that you too can be truly present in the spirit, able to connect without words. Use touch, eye contact, music, aroma – and try to breach the barrier of communication between us. Look into our eyes and look for that spark that may alight when you connect. You are creating within us a moment of wellbeing – by the end of the day, with a string of such moments, we will feel good, even if we do not know why.

Try to realize that it is not important that we remember that you visited us, for it is the experience of Christ's love that you bring us, not a memory of an event. Ask yourself: why do you want us to remember that you came? If we have enjoyed your visit at the time, does it matter that a few hours later we will have forgotten that you have given of yourself and brought the Christ-light to us?

Is dementia a gift?

Live intensely in the present.

Inner spirit is revealed.

Connect spirit to spirit.

As we lose identity in the world around us, we are who we are, a person created in the image of God.

Our spiritual self is given meaning as a transcendent being.

We live intensely in the present moment, so do not have that sense of a time just past. Is this not what Jesus asks of us all? Maybe dementia can be reframed as a gift, because we are enabled by our deficits to live only in the present moment, apart from glimpses of the recent past and some intense video clips of our more distant past.

As we lose an identity in the world around us, which is so anxious to define us by what we do or say, rather than who we are, we can seek an identity by simply being who we are, a person created in the image of God. Our spiritual self is reflected in the divine and given meaning as a transcendent being. As our cognition fades and our emotions flatten, our spirituality can flourish as an important source of identity.

Our spirit remains deep within, despite the ravages of dementia. We can connect spirit to spirit, even at the last stages. Indeed, I have seen such true connection occur. You need to breach the barrier between us, which is created by a society that places such value on cognition.

As time passes, we will need others to understand and realize that our odd behaviour, our lack of social graces, our lack of resources to offer in friendship, do not stem from our soul within. Rather, they are simply the result of our damaged brain. You will need to be able to see past our confusion to relate to our soul, and to see us as God sees us all, as His children.

Minister to us

Our relationship with God needs your increasing support.

Sing with us, pray for us.

Trust in Him to help you to connect with our soul.

Let us live through your memories, as ours become unreliable and fragmented. Never let it be that we should say, 'My God, My God, why have you forsaken me?' You can walk alongside us as we approach the valley of the shadow of death.

As we travel this journey of dissolution, our relationship with God needs increasing support from you, our fellowship in the body of Christ. Don't abandon us at any stage, for the Holy Spirit connects us, linking our souls, not our minds or brains. Please don't exclude us from our normal spiritual practices, as we need to receive nurture to our spirit as we approach death from dementia.

We need you to minister to us, to sing with us and to pray for us, to be our memory for us. The liturgy, familiar hymns or choruses, the Lord's Prayer, these are ways in which you can help us join with you in our walk with God.

We might become agitated or don't understand, so tap into the rich resources of the Holy Spirit and remember that you are connecting with our soul, not our brain. Be creative and trust in God to help you to connect with us at this eternal level. The Trinity can be a model for our relationship in pastoral care. Through the power of the Holy Spirit, we are in communion with each other and with God. There is no need for cognition, for this is a spiritual communion.

Communion with Triune God

Joining you in worship in spirit and in truth.

We connect with the Christ-light around us in fellowship.

We feel God's everlasting arms beneath us.

'Remember me when you come into your kingdom.'

We may forget God, but He never forgets us.

Worship is in spirit and truth, not in cognition, and we are in communion with the Triune God, whose nature is to be in relationship.

What about the Eucharist? The sacrament is 'an effectual sign of grace by which He works invisibly in us'. Why should our lack of memory deny us this sign of grace?

I believe those without the ability to remember are a sacred part of this Eucharistic meal. The thief said to Jesus, 'Remember me when you come into your kingdom.'

We may forget God, but He never forgets us. He holds us in the palm of His hand even through the dissolution of dementia.

Will I know God if I can no longer remember? In my first book I write:

> As I unfold before God, as this disease unwraps me, opens up the treasures of what lies within my multi-fold personality, I can feel safe as each layer is gently opened out. God's everlasting arms will be beneath me, upholding me.

As we lose our memory of who we are and who God is, we can become reflected in others and see Christ in others. In the family of God, the body of Christ, we are what others remember of us, and we connect with the Christ-light around us in fellowship.

You need to shine the Christ-light for us, to affirm our identity and to walk alongside us in our confusion. We may not be able to affirm you, to remember who you are or whether you have visited us, but you have represented Christ's remembrance to us.

Reframe dementia

Journeying into a state of unknowing.

Barriers of cognition and emotion being stripped away to reveal spirit deep within.

Forgetting and losing our self, we are finding the presence of God.

Stripped naked before God, journeying towards a deepening I–Thou relationship.

This journey – from diagnosis to death from dementia – is a journey into the true centre of our being – our spirit deep within. Our soul remains, despite the ravages of dementia causing the brain to become diseased and die.

Do our diminished communication and less reliable emotions mean our spirit is disappearing? I do not believe this is the case, even though we might have trouble feeling the presence of God and speaking the words of prayers out loud or in our mind. Still we can commune with the divine without words.

Our soul is given life and meaning in our Christian community. You play a vital role in relating to the soul within us, connecting at this eternal level. Reassure us of your presence and, through you, Christ's presence.

Let's reframe the experience of dementia as a journey into a state of unknowing, towards a deepening I–Thou relationship, where the barriers of cognition and emotion are being stripped away to reveal an intensely present spirit deep within. We are being stripped naked before God, as were Adam and Eve before eating of the Tree of the Knowledge of Good and Evil.

Forgetting and losing our self, through you we can find the presence of God. By reframing the experience of dementia in this way, it may help you in your pastoral outreach to those of us with dementia.

All are made in God's image

God sees our heart and our spirit.

His Spirit connects us to Him and each other.

Be alongside, helping us to find meaning.

Welcome outcasts and minister to us.

Hold out the Christ-light to us.

Reframe your view of dementia, reflect on what it means to be truly human and in relationship with the Triune God.

Never forget that God sees our heart and our spirit, not our mind or body. We are fearfully and wonderfully formed in the image of God. The breath of life given to us – the Holy Spirit – draws our spirit deeper into relationship with the divine and with each other.

As chaplains, you can travel alongside us on our journey, helping us to find meaning and purpose in life. It will be challenging to see beyond our cognitive and emotional deficits, but do what Jesus did, welcoming the outcasts and ministering to them. Simply be alongside us, include us and surround us in Christ's love. You can show us the beacon of hope, by holding the Christ-light for us, drawing us ever closer into the I–Thou.

By reframing your understanding of dementia, you have a chance to reflect on what it means to be truly human and to be in relationship with the Triune God.

Thank you.

INDEX

NOTHING ABOUT US, WITHOUT US!

NOTHING ABOUT US, WITHOUT US!